MIND AND MUSCLE

Mind and Muscle

an owner's handbook

by

Elizabeth Langford

drawings by

Enci Noro

Foreword by Walter Carrington

Garant

Leuven-Apeldoorn

First print: 1999
Second print: 2001

Elizabeth Langford
Mind and Muscle
An Owner's Handbook
Leuven / Apeldoorn:
Garant
First print: 1999
xvi + 253 pp., 24 cm
D/1999/5779/67
ISBN 90-5350-883-X
NUGI 752

Drawings: Enci Noro
Cover design: Danni Elskens

Published by Garant Uitgevers N.V.
Somersstraat 13-15, B-2018 Antwerpen, Belgium
Koninginnelaan 96, NL-7315 EB/Apeldoorn, Holland
e-mail: uitgeverij@garant.be

A WORD ABOUT THE TITLE

When you buy a car, or other sophisticated equipment, you are likely to receive two handbooks. One you will probably never look at – it belongs to the realm of servicing and repairs by experts. The other contains just the information that you need in order to use the equipment appropriately. You will never buy any equipment as sophisticated as your own nerves and muscles – the system by which you move. Here, then, is the owner's manual you never received.

Our bodies are influenced by our suppositions about them: hence the paramount importance of getting the facts straight, of uprooting misconceptions. To this end, the book gathers together essential information not previously accessible to the general reader. It covers what is, for many people, an unfamiliar area of knowledge – and does so in such a way as to render that knowledge available for practical, everyday use.

In a book with 'muscle' in its title, you might expect to find *exercises*... but not in this one. Here, on the other hand, you will find *experiments* to carry out for yourself; they are designed to reveal how intimately mind and muscle are linked – far more so than most people imagine. As explanation unfolds, these experiments, taken in sequence, form a practical guide enabling the reader to set aside hearsay, while verifying facts from personal experience. In this way many costly mistakes can be avoided.

This approach raises questions that many people have never asked. They may not have asked the questions because at some time they were fed the wrong answers; or because, in daily life, the essential link between theory and practice can be hard to find. Knowledge, acquired as an adult, often finds itself at odds with long-standing physical habits rooted in misconceptions dating from early childhood. Theory, if lodged in the intellect without reaching the muscles, is less than useful to someone who is in pain – or who meets obstacles in the way of artistic or athletic development, for example.

This type of difficulty requires, for its solution, an awareness, not only of habitual muscular patterns, but also of the background thinking with which they are associated. It calls for the identification of assumptions, conscious or otherwise, which cause unnecessary problems. The present book, based on the author's long teaching experience in this field, is offered as a practical guide to the improved use of mind and muscle.

CONTENTS

PART VII   DISCOVERING THE MAP

LIST OF ILLUSTRATIONS

ACKNOWLEDGEMENTS

I should like to thank Walter Carrington for writing the foreword to this book – a great honour. My thanks to him, and to my other teachers, especially Peggy Williams, must at least be recorded here: I am at a loss to express them adequately. Nor have I words for the pleasure I take in Enci Noro's drawings, an integral part of what the book is intended to convey.

Ted Dimon, president of the Alexander Technique Archives, Inc., gave permission to reproduce 'Startle Pattern' photographs from F.P. Jones's *Method for changing stereotyped response patterns by the inhibition of certain postural sets*. The reactions derived from 'Startle Pattern' were perceptively mimed by Alain d'Ursel, and skilfully photographed by Athanase Vettas. I am grateful to all three for this important contribution, as well as to Athanase Vettas for his many other photographs reproduced here. Clare Hughes took the photographs which, with her kind permission, are shown here as figs. 35 and 42. I regret that I have been unable to trace the copyright holder of the newspaper photograph reproduced in Chapter 2. The stanza from 'i thank You God for most this amazing' is reprinted from COMPLETE POEMS 1904–1962, by E.E. Cummings, edited by George J. Firmage, by permission of W.W. Norton & Company, Copyright © 1991 by the Trustees for the E.E. Cummings Trust and George James Firmage.

The late Ann Fletcher saw the early chapters, and urged me to write the book she 'had always wanted to read'. I hope Malcolm King knows the extent to which his enthusiasm helped me to sustain the impetus needed to finish it. My profound thanks are also due to Monique Vanormelingen for much painstaking work in preparing the text for publication.

FOREWORD

Betty Langford is a gifted professional musician, but she is also an experienced teacher of the F. Matthias Alexander Technique. I can vouch for her skill and knowledge because she trained in our school many years ago and has remained a colleague and a steadfast friend. Her teaching experience has led her to a clear insight into the needs of her pupils and particularly their need for more information than is ordinarily to be derived from individual lessons in the Technique. It has also led her to the conviction that such information can and should be made more widely available. Hence the publication of this book.

F. Matthias Alexander himself was a singular exponent of the Delphic injunction, *Know Thyself*. His Technique was the outcome of long and painstaking self-experiment through which he gained a vast amount of practical experience and knowledge. He wrote four books to describe what he had done: and when anybody sought an interview with him, they would be asked immediately whether they had read any of them. If not, they were requested to do so before an appointment could be made.

However, Alexander's books, invaluable in themselves, are not concerned with ordinary information about anatomy and physiology and related topics: they deal with the practicalities of the Technique, and many students ever since have felt the need for more general information, presented in a way that can be directly related to practical studies. From her own long experience of study and research, Betty has been able to supply this need to a very satisfactory extent and I therefore commend this book to all who would wish to follow in Alexander's footsteps.

Walter Carrington
London, 20th August, 1998

PART I
ESTABLISHING THE CONTEXT

CHAPTER 1

TOWARDS A SENSE OF DIRECTION

> I may seem to stress too much the preoccupation of the
> brain with muscle. Can we stress too much that preoccu-
> pation when any path we trace in the brain leads directly
> or indirectly to muscle?
>
> Sir Charles Sherrington *The Brain and its Mechanism*

Throughout history, it seems, there have always been people who sought a clearer awareness of themselves and how they relate to the world. Their quest has varied in emphasis:
at times the stress has been religious, at others it has been variously philosophical, politi-
cal, psychological. A characteristic of our own time is a feeling that the search is incomplete if it does not take into account our nature as physical creatures who have to live in
and with our own bodies. This awareness is by no means new, but it has acquired a renewed urgency for a generation that relies less and less on its own physical energy for the
work that has to be done. What is this body, sometimes so weary that even thinking
about it seems tedious, sometimes bursting with a superfluous energy that is in itself a
burden because it lacks a sufficient outlet?

It is not surprising that there is much searching and a vast explosion of fashionable
techniques and systems for exercising and for increasing physical awareness. How satisfied are we with the results of all this surge of interest? Where is it getting us, if anywhere? Could our seeking be given a more reliable sense of direction?

This book is my attempt to answer the last question. It draws on my thirty years' experience as an Alexander teacher – but it is not intended as yet another introduction to
the Alexander Technique. (See Chapter 34.) What prompts me to write is the fact that, in
the course of teaching people from most walks of life and many countries, I have come
to recognize the extent and the danger of widespread misconceptions about the relationship between mind and muscle.

There has come into being what I may call a pseudo-scientific folk-lore that is in itself a source of problems. Creeping misinformation is rampant. Unfounded statements
are repeated so often – in print and by word of mouth – that many, perhaps most people
take their truth for granted. And few can have the time to challenge this body of pseudo-
knowledge, to check it by comparison with known and verifiable facts – for these are
most often expressed in technical terminology and smothered in more information than

5

the general reader wants or needs.

F.M. Alexander maintained that, provided we can avoid fundamental errors in the way we use ourselves, 'the right thing does itself'. As he showed, the human organism is indeed self-regulating to an amazing extent – BUT ... nobody can afford to forget that proviso! I hope in this book to clear away some fundamental mistakes which block the self-regulating process.

The planned sequence of the book seeks first of all to do away with misconceptions. Then follows some clarification of facts and of the terms used to discuss them. After this comes a series of experiments; I hope you will use them to check my explanations for yourself. All this is important in paving the way for more specific advice later in the book, for I do not think it wise to follow suggestions without understanding the thinking behind them. In this way, each chapter prepares what follows, so I hope that, after perhaps leafing through to get a general idea of the contents, the reader will then turn to the beginning and read the book in sequence. On a first reading, the cross-references will indicate where threads from one chapter will be picked up in another. Later, the cross-references will be seen to be a vital part of the book, for the greatest benefit is to be obtained from its continuous use for an ever-deepening understanding of the subject – which is of course, yourself.

This is not a book for anyone with a dislike of questioning received ideas; nor is it a collection of easy recipes. Despite the non-technical language – and the occasional note of frivolity – this is a serious book. A great neurologist has said that 'any path we trace in the brain leads ... to muscle' and I believe that a practical handbook about this relationship will be of use to those who like thinking things through and who enjoy their own capacity to use both mind and muscle.

CHAPTER 2

HOW THIS BOOK CAME TO BE WRITTEN
A PERSONAL STORY

'Her ladyship wishes you to convey it to its destination
personally, realising that, should she entrust it to the ordinary channels, the gift will be delayed in its arrival beyond
the essential date.'
'You mean, if she posts it, it won't get there in time?'

P.G. Wodehouse *Joy in the Morning*

When I was young, it would have been useful to me had I had a book, written in plain
language and aimed at removing misunderstandings about mind and muscle. I was,
even more than most people, a victim of misinformation, for I began to learn the violin
at the age of three – and unfortunately the teaching I received was unsound, both technically and physiologically. Even without photographic evidence (figs. 1–9) it would be
clear to me now that my early development was impeded in this way. As a music student, and later as a professional violinist, the more I worked, the more I suffered physically from basic faults that a conventional musical training did nothing to rectify. Nevertheless, because I like music – and because it was how I earned my living – I struggled
on, usually in pain and often frustrated by my inability to play as well as I wanted to.

When I was thirty, I went to a great violin teacher, the late Max Rostal, and asked his
help in rebuilding my technique from the ground up. His clear view of my difficulties
enabled me to place my approach to the instrument on a much more rational footing.
But by then, as Rostal himself recognized, I also had other problems, outside the scope
of any violin teacher. As Rostal put it, 'You have understood my technique – what worries me is your posture.' Later, I came to understand what this really meant: that not
only my playing but all my activity was based on a way of managing my body that was
unsatisfactory. Despite this, my playing improved, which led to greater professional demands on me – and eventually to a crisis.

While I was sub-leader (second concertmaster) of the Royal Liverpool Philharmonic
Orchestra, the long series of minor aches and pains culminated in back pain so appalling
that I was helpless, even dependent on friends to turn me over in bed. Fortunately, I had
a profound certainty that this trouble had not fallen on me out of nowhere but that I
was myself in some way the cause of it, and that this was why both medical and osteo-
pathic help had proved ineffective. My problem was in fact wear and tear rather than illness; milder forms than mine were, as I knew, commonplace among musicians – long

before Repetitive Strain Injury hit the headlines – so the idea was not unfamiliar to me. (I have since been able to understand just how and why this had happened to me.)

Performing musicians have to think quite a lot about how they do things. They try other ways, take lessons, are used to the idea that they may be quite mistaken in how they are going about something. So it was natural to me to look for someone who could tell me where I had gone wrong. By taking Alexander lessons, I learned to question my most basic assumptions about how to do very ordinary things: sitting, standing, walking, picking things up, raising my arms. Gradually I acquired the background understanding that I had always lacked, and started applying it to the more complex task of playing the violin. This was to prove fruitful: ever since, when preparing and performing demanding programmes, I have done so without a twinge. Of course, at first I had to set aside some long-standing habits, and revise some of my received ideas. The mess I was in at the time left me in no doubt about the need for this.

What I was learning interested me extremely and I wanted to be able to share it. I was already having Alexander lessons with Walter Carrington; now he accepted me for training as an Alexander teacher. I felt fortunate in having come as near to the source as it was possible to get: during the last years of Alexander's life, Walter had been his principal assistant, in charge of the training of teachers. The three-year full-time course left me much better informed and keen to understand the difficulties of people who came to me for Alexander lessons.

At first, I had expected to be working mainly with musicians. In the event, I have always found myself teaching all sorts of people, for their personal well-being, whatever their activity in life: actors and artists; barristers and businessmen; convalescents and computer programmers; dancers, dentists, diplomats, doctors; economists, farmers, gardeners, housewives, interpreters; jugglers, lecturers, mime artists, nurses; osteopaths and psychologists; riding instructors, schoolteachers, secretaries, teachers of Tai Chi Chuan and translators, waiters, Yoga teachers, zoologists – and many more. I have given lessons to a Chelsea Pensioner and to a multi-millionaire; to athletes and to handicapped children; I have taught physiotherapists and their patients, and given individual lessons to a community of nuns. The youngest person I ever taught was a handicapped four-year-old who didn't make eye contact – it was a great day when he peered into my face, saying 'How you've aged since last time!' And I remember a woman of eighty saying, 'I want to continue perfect until the end.' It has all been – and still is – a tremendous learning process for me, too.

Despite all this variety, the work with musicians has always been important. Soon after I qualified as an Alexander teacher, Allen Percival, then Principal of the Guildhall School of Music, gave me the opportunity of doing pioneer work in setting up courses in the Alexander Technique as part of the normal G.S.M. curriculum. The following year, Sir William Glock invited me to teach and lecture at the international Summer School for music at Dartington. Other leading music schools soon followed the Guildhall's example; in a number of countries, access to Alexander lessons is now regarded as usual in the training of musicians. It is pleasant to see this progress, though it seems that there is still some way to go before the Alexander work and other studies are sufficiently integrated. My best experiences of the kind of integration I have in mind have been in collaboration with the pianist Rudolf Kratzert and the singer Malcolm King, both of whom are also Alexander teachers.

At the time I received my STAT diploma[1], the few teacher training courses then in existence were directed by former pupils of F.M. Alexander himself. I had the honour of being the first of the second generation of Alexander teachers to be authorized by STAT to run my own school. When one trains Alexander teachers, one has at least three years in which to get to know them and to make sure not only of their competence but of their understanding of the principles involved. However, in the rest of my teaching practice (i.e. when working with people who come for shorter periods, to learn for themselves and not in order to become teachers) I noticed that pupils were not always aware of the implications of the improvements they experienced, and so were less well protected from misinformation than they might have been. I also started thinking about people who don't have Alexander lessons, but who might well be better off without some of the mistaken ideas that surround us, and to which anyone can easily fall prey.

Then I thought that Alexander's emphasis on not misusing physical mechanisms might usefully be extended to questioning the beliefs and assumptions responsible for misuse. This questioning was implicit in the Alexander Technique as I had been taught it, but there did not seem to be a book written on just those lines, so I decided to write one. The gestation period has been long, but this causes me no regret, for it has given me a chance to test the usefulness of what I have written. Successive drafts were tried out on pupils and friends – the whole undertaking owes much to their questions, criticisms and encouragement.

---

1. The Society of Teachers of the Alexander Technique (STAT) is London-based, with a world-wide membership; a number of countries have their own societies which are affiliated to STAT. I served on the council of STAT for some thirteen years (for two of them as chairman) and now train Alexander teachers in Belgium.

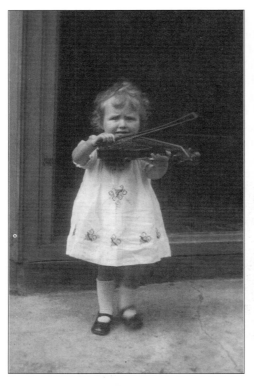

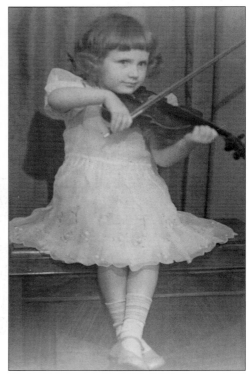

— Fig. 1 —
I began to learn the violin at the age of three...

— Fig. 2 —
... but the teaching I received was unsound, both technically and physiologically.

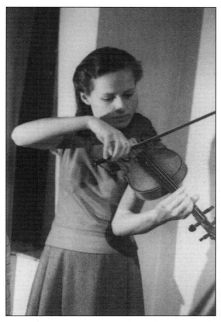

— *Fig. 3* —

... the more I worked, the more I suffered physically...

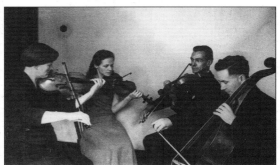

— *Fig. 4* —

... because I like music... I struggled on...

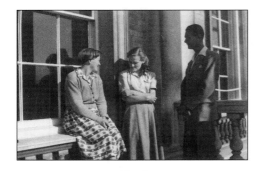

— *Fig. 5* —

This posture was typical of me at the time.

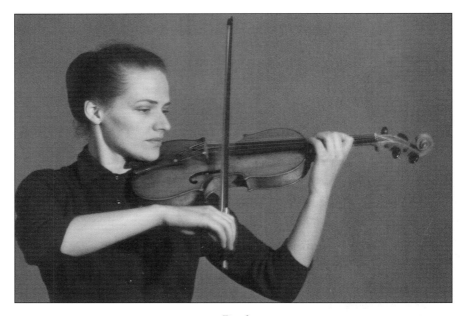

— Fig. 6 —

... Rostal said 'You have understood my technique... but...

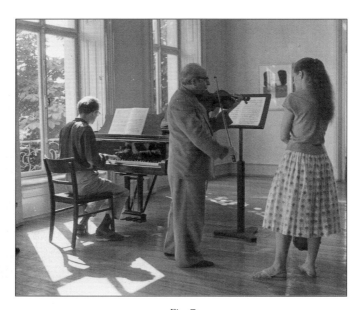

— Fig. 7 —

... what worries me is your posture.'

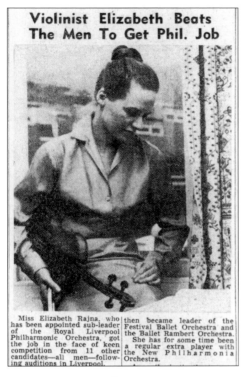

Violinist Elizabeth Beats The Men To Get Phil. Job

Miss Elizabeth Rajna, who has been appointed sub-leader of the Royal Liverpool Philharmonic Orchestra, got the job in the face of keen competition from 11 other candidates—all men—following auditions in Liverpool. then became leader of the Festival Ballet Orchestra and the Ballet Rambert Orchestra. She has for some time been a regular extra player with the New Philharmonia Orchestra.

— *Fig. 8* —

Greater professional demands ... led to a crisis, publicity surrounding the – then highly unusual – appointment having added to the stress...

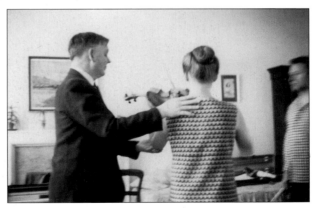

— *Fig. 9* —

... acquired background understanding, and started applying it... (an Alexander lesson with Walter Carrington)

PART II
CLEARING THE DECKS

CHAPTER 3

MOVEMENT AND THE BODY-IMAGE

... 'body-image' may be the first mental construct and self-construct there is, the one that acts as a model for all others...

Oliver Sacks *A Leg to Stand On*

Everyone reading this will have some preconceived ideas about the human body – ideas accumulated with or without conscious study. It seems to me natural that this should be so, for the body is a fact we can hardly ignore.

Starting in early childhood, we build a mental picture made up of two views of ourselves: 1) from outside, what we look like – mixed perhaps with what we wish we looked like – and 2) from inside, the continuous stream of feelings and sensations that tell us where we are and how we are, and which supply us with feedback confirming that we are doing what we intend. We are not always aware of this flow of information, but life would be difficult without it. Remember trying to drink without dribbling when the dentist has given you an anaesthetic? Remember the insecurity of stepping on a foot that has 'gone to sleep'?

This mental picture of ourselves is also influenced by our perception of the world around us: observation of other people, of dolls and mechanical toys, of how things in general balance and function – for we sense that we ourselves are subject to the same mechanical laws, the same gravitational force.

Then, too, there are the ideas that present themselves as we go along, things people tell us, things we read: information (not necessarily reliable) about how this body of ours is 'put together', how it works, exhortations about posture, exercise, breathing, relaxation and so on. In the haphazard way of children, we absorb some or all of this and add it to the mental picture we are building.

Thus, before we have any opportunity to study the question consciously, indeed before developing our capacity for critical appraisal of information, we are already in possession of a rag-bag of ideas, of which some may indeed correspond to the facts. On the other hand, mixed with these may well be half-truths, guess-work and some over-compensation for previous misunderstandings. There may even be a certain amount of sheer superstition.

How important is it to be well-informed in this respect? If it were possible to be totally innocent of any conscious mental image of our own bodies, perhaps we should get along all right – I am not sure. What I do know for certain is that, in this domain, misconceptions are dangerous and tend to be self-perpetuating. For what I have seen again and again, in thirty years of practical teaching, is that the way people move is governed by what they suppose their bodies to be – by their personal body-image. Consciously or otherwise, this body-image is with us all the time, influencing every movement we make, whatever we happen to be doing: at work, at play, in every activity from the most mundane task to the most demanding exercise of skill. It also affects the way we keep still and the way we do what we call 'relaxing'. It even makes itself felt in our moods, our thinking, our capacity for learning. Movements which go against the true nature of the organism lead to unacceptable wear and tear. Hence, if this body-image contains positive inaccuracies, it is dangerous to well-being.

My purpose in writing this book is not to try to tell you 'all about your body'. No one person could do that. If such a study interests you, there are many fine textbooks on anatomy and physiology already in existence for those with patience and a good many years to spare. There is so much information! The problem, as so often in our society, is one of distribution, of bringing the relevant bits of knowledge together 'at the sharp end' where they are needed in daily life. How can we be expected to take a responsible attitude to ourselves if the necessary minimum of information is not readily available to us?

There are plenty of things for which we all can and do accept responsibility, without being experts: whoever would send for an electrician to change a light bulb, or for a tailor to sew on a button? If your sink gets blocked, you don't instantly assume that the plumbing is faulty, you guess that something unsuitable has gone down the plug-hole. Was it carelessness or was the sink-tidy missing? And where is the thing for unblocking the sink? For good management of ourselves, the information we need is often on that mundane level – information seriously lacking in most people's education.

We cannot all be expected to know as much anatomical detail as a surgeon, nor do we need it. Not everyone who drives a car needs to be an expert motor mechanic – but I remember an experienced mechanic telling me that whenever he serviced a car he had a pretty good idea of how it had been driven. What would happen if the only people who knew how to drive a car properly were the top racing drivers? This is roughly analogous to the present state of knowledge about our own locomotor system! Some (not all) fine athletes, dancers, and performing musicians know very well what they are doing with their bodies. The rest of humanity is quite surprisingly vague about something that concerns us all so intimately, accepting it as a matter of luck whether things go wrong or not.

If you doubt this, ask yourself why what is vaguely known as 'backache' or 'back pain' is the most common ailment after the common cold. At a time when industrial action was regarded as a major problem in Britain, backache, which has since increased dramatically, was already responsible for at least three times as many lost working days as were lost through strikes (1980 statistics). More recently, not only has 'Repetitive Strain Injury' been recognized by the British Courts, but its abbreviation, 'RSI', has come to be part of the language. The symptoms are very real and painful, but I feel that to regard it simply as an 'illness' does little to dispel confusion surrounding the root causes. (**See Chapter 30.**)

All this is not because doctors are falling down on the job: many of the people concerned are not 'ill' in the usual sense of the word. But it is not their own fault, either; nor are they malingering. The fact is that they are suffering from wear and tear resulting from a mistaken body-image. I have heard doctors avow that in such cases, whatever the treatment, the patient will soon be back again, because even the wonders of modern medicine and surgery cannot be expected to compete with this constant wear and tear. Even more alarming, such problems are no longer exclusively associated with the ageing process – more and more young people are becoming affected. (**Some historical and social reasons for this are discussed in Chapters 18 and 33.**)

A faulty body-image leaves people prey to all sorts of nonsense; to old wives' tales, to magazine articles written by journalists without specialized knowledge, to well-meaning but ill-informed advice from family, friends and teachers, to the influence of admired public figures who may not necessarily be good models to imitate, to fashionable crazes for unsuitable types of exercise, and so on. There are even ways of standing and sitting that have more to do with fashion than with common sense or comfort (fig. 10). A body-image based securely on fact is a necessary defence against these and similar influences.

A well-founded body-image also helps us to avoid having – however unwittingly – a negative influence on other people. We are all imitative creatures, children particularly so. It seems to me that each of us has a social responsibility to avoid polluting the environment with bad example and ill-informed advice.

So what I hope to do throughout this book is to clear away some misunderstandings I often encounter in the course of teaching people how they can move more efficiently. The information I shall give may not necessarily fit in with ideas you already hold or with what you have been told up to now, but I am sure it is consistent with what is so far known about the workings of our bodies. In the hope that you will check up on what I say, I have given reasons and references wherever possible – otherwise, why should you believe me more than anyone else? A healthy scepticism is the best defence against all the people (including me) who try to tell others what to do![1]

In 1966, when I began seriously to study the subject of human movement, I had no theoretical knowledge at all, so I understand only too well that many of my readers have neither the time nor the inclination to learn a technical vocabulary. For this reason I have used everyday language where possible, on the grounds that something we use every day (as indeed we are obliged to use our bodies) must be capable of being discussed in those terms. This is too important a matter to be left to 'experts' – and in fact there is no way of doing so!

There is one effort that I do want to ask of the reader, for the sake of avoiding confusion. It is the mental effort of setting aside his or her existing body-image for long enough to question the assumptions, conscious or otherwise, on which it is founded.

---

1. From the date of some of the references, you may well conclude that facts, however well established, and however relevant to daily life, can often take an amazing time to find general acceptance.

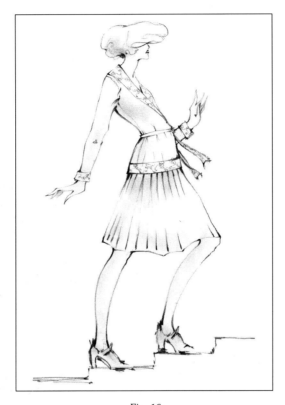

_ *Fig. 10* _

A fashion design – but not a good model to imitate

Chapter 4

SOME COMMON ERRORS IN THE BODY-IMAGE

The man who can tell me where I am wrong is my friend
for life.

F.M. Alexander

Let me explain a bit more about the way a faulty body-image affects the way we use ourselves. In this chapter I shall quote examples of some of the mistakes I have come across
all too frequently. I shall begin each example by giving you the opportunity to check
your own body-image against the facts. Please answer each question very quickly, without stopping to think – that is the way to find out what assumptions you are making as
you go about your daily life. Indeed, you may find that these *assumptions* (revealed by
your first reaction) bear little relation to any actual *knowledge* you have. (See the case of
the doctor, below.) Please don't feel silly if this happens. This is not a moment for
bothering about intellectual pride. Nor is this a school test – it is not important to 'get
the right answer'. It is seriously important to you to know on what basis you are using
your own body.

1) ***Where is your hip-joint?*** Please put your hand on the place where you think it is – at
once! Now stop and think. Is that really the place where the leg is 'hinged' on the body?
Experiment and make sure. Now have a look at fig. 12. Never mind if you were mistaken – be glad you found out! Lots of people get this one wrong, probably because they
have heard the expression 'hands on hips', meaning as in fig. 11. But that is the top of
the hip-bone; the joint is much lower, as you realize once you think about it and try to
move the leg independently of other bony structures.

I once put the same question individually to every pupil in a school for gifted children aged 8 to 18 – and got only one correct answer. So I was not particularly surprised
to find that the walking problems of a distinguished lawyer were due to the same error in
his body-image. Once he understood where the hip-joint really is, the 'stiffness' that was
troubling him simply disappeared – so much so that he could thoroughly enjoy running
regularly in the woods with his dog, not so much for the sake of exercise as for the sheer
pleasure of moving as nature intended.

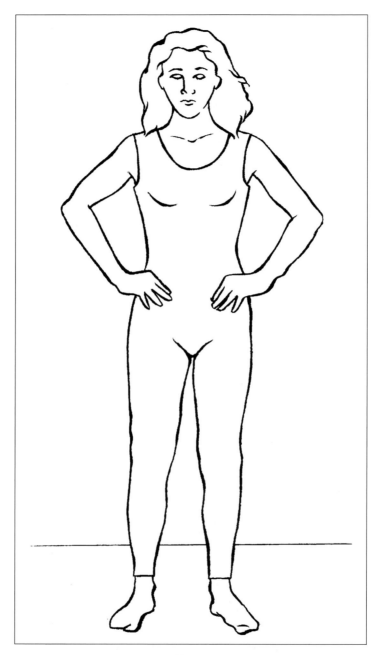

— *Fig. 11* —
Where is your hip-joint? *Not* here!

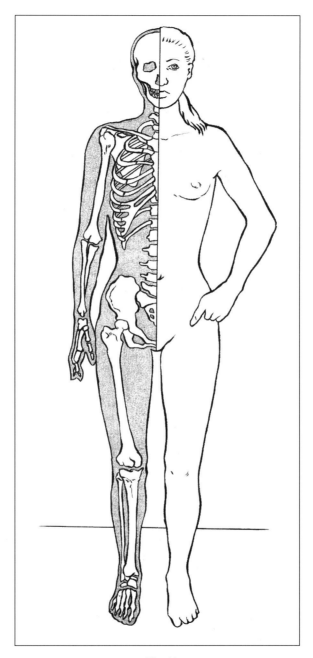

— Fig. 12 —

This is were the hip-joint is.

23

You see, if you suppose, even subconsciously, that your legs are joined to your body somewhere near waist level, it is from there that you will try to move them – which means that you will almost inevitably start each step by an ill-advised movement of your pelvis, instead of letting your leg swing freely from its real joint. Not only does this limit leg movement, it is also bad for your lower back. **(See Chapter 21.)**

2) *Where is the joint between your head and your spine?* Point quickly, as before. Most people place this joint much too low. Even those who think of it at the right height usually place it too far back. Fig. 13 shows where it really is: approximately between your ears. **(See also fig. 24, Chapter 14.)**

Does that surprise you? I doubt if you are as surprised as a doctor who came to see me a few years ago, explaining in precise technical language the trouble he was having with his back. All the time he was talking, I was wondering if the way he held his head might be a contributing factor to his back pain. After a while I said:

'However much a person knows about anatomy, that knowledge sometimes remains, as it were, outside him. Even a doctor can, so to speak, leave his knowledge on the printed page or in the patient's body, failing to include it in his personal body image. He can continue to use his own body on the basis of ideas acquired in childhood; the habit built up at that time remains untouched by knowledge acquired later. So now show me, please, without stopping to think, where is your *atlanto-occipital* joint?' (technical name of the joint in question).

The doctor immediately touched a point about halfway down the back of his neck – then burst out laughing as his anatomical knowledge caught up with that first reaction (which was, as I had guessed, rooted in a body-image dating from early childhood). He then quickly understood that, since in this body-image the real joint was *assumed not to exist*, he was holding it stiff to correspond with the image – and only allowing himself to move from lower down, which had its problems. Worse still, the fact that he was assuming the joint to be not only much *lower*, but also *further back* than it really is, meant (according to his body-image) that the weight of his head had no central support. No wonder he felt the need to hold on to it tightly! And it was this persistent holding on tight at the back of the neck which turned out to be indirectly responsible for the pain in his back.

A word of warning: if you think you have been making a similar mistake, I strongly advise you *not to try to correct it immediately*. To do so might well mean jumping out of the frying-pan into the fire. **(This is explained in Chapter 10.)** Head balance is crucial to the well-being of the whole person, so we shall return to it in more detail **(in Chapters 13 to 17)**. Please be patient until then.

3) *Where is your diaphragm?* Most people know that they have something called a diaphragm which is somehow important in breathing. But it is really astonishing how many people are ready to hand out advice on 'diaphragmatic breathing' when they have actually no idea, or a wrong idea, of where this precious diaphragm is to be found. It is even more amazing how many people listen to them!

Did you think the diaphragm was that bit between your ribs in front, above your navel? If not, I apologise to you – but I have come across innumerable intelligent people who thought just that, and who therefore imagined that they were doing a good thing by making themselves bulge there when breathing in.

If you knew that it is in fact a muscle inside your ribcage, where you can neither see nor touch it, a sort of two-domed ceiling to the abdomen, separating the abdominal organs from the heart and lungs – good. But at what level do you picture it? (Fig. 14) Did you realize how high it is in front (attaching itself to the inside of the lower part of the breastbone) and that, inside you, parts of it are higher still some of the time? Do you know how low it is joined at the back? (Fig. 18, Chapter 11) Trace on your own body the shape of your lowest ribs (not forgetting the small 'floating' ribs.) The diaphragm is attached to the bottom six ribs, and goes all the way round from breastbone to spine, where it is attached to most of the lumbar vertebrae, i.e. it joins the inside of your spine in the small of your back. Of course, because of breathing, the whole thing is in constant movement – but did you know that the diaphragm never flattens out completely but retains its shape (something like a rather odd umbrella) during breathing movements? (Those nature films of swimming jellyfish can help us to form a rough picture.) More about the diaphragm later. (Chapter 11) Here we are just clearing the decks, so to speak.

I could give many examples of physical problems resulting from mental muddles of this kind. Shall I tell you about the girl who thought her ribs were fixed (i.e. not hinged) to her spine? No wonder she was obliged to breathe by lifting and dropping her chest – a very tiring and inefficient procedure. Or I could tell you about a violinist who thought to settle a technical argument by saying 'In any case, when you move your left arm into the playing position, your shoulder just naturally accompanies it up and forward.' Well, *his* shoulder did, because he had forgotten the existence of the shoulder joint – and that meant a grave limitation on the freedom of his arm.

A student of mine once asked fifty five-year-olds to draw themselves without clothes: every child drew a horizontal line at waist level! Amusing, yes, but not if it leads them to suppose that there is a real division there, an idea that easily encourages an inappropriate amount of bending in that part of the body, with consequent back trouble later on. (See Chapters 19, 22, 23.)

Building up for yourself a body-image that corresponds to the facts is rather like putting together a jigsaw puzzle: until you have put quite a few bits together, it is hard to see what the total picture is likely to be. That is why I shall keep on asking you to be patient, for I should be very sorry if anyone were to jump to wrong conclusions through reacting too quickly to what is in this book.

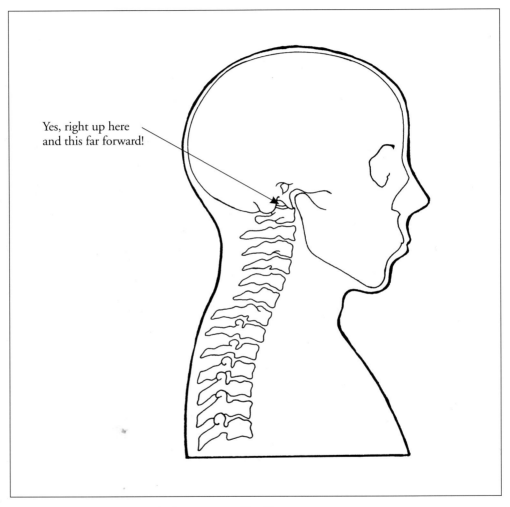

Yes, right up here
and this far forward!

— *Fig. 13* —

Where is the joint between your head and the top of your spine?

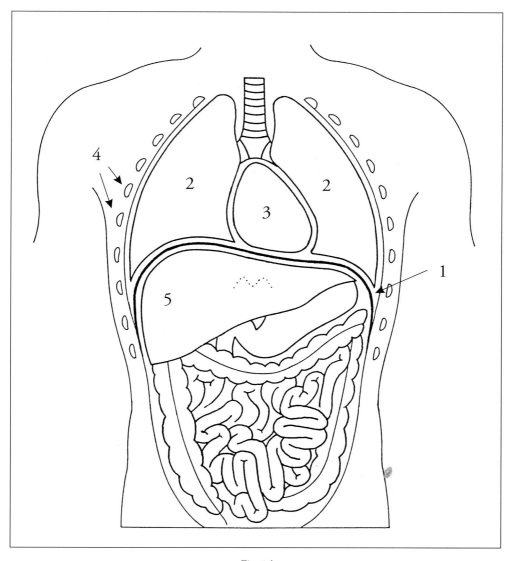

— *Fig. 14* —

Where is your diaphragm? The diaphragm separates abdominal organs from heart and lungs.
(Sectional diagram: 1. thick black line represents the diaphragm; 2. lungs; 3. heart; 4. ribs; 5. liver. Dotted line shows level of tip of breast-bone.)

CHAPTER 5

AN ETERNAL TRIANGLE

Life is a desperate struggle to succeed in being in fact what
we are in design.
Ortega y Gasset

The body-image of which we have spoken in the previous chapters has several aspects:
1) *What the body is:* the materials from which it is made up; the way the various parts
   are put together; its shape; i.e. its **Structure**.
2) *The way the body works:* how it performs its various operations (breathing, circulation, digestion, etc.); the way it moves (the action of muscles on joints and so forth);
   i.e. its **Functioning**. (I make a distinction between *function* and *functioning*: it is the
   function of my car to take me from A to B; if something is not quite right with its
   functioning, it may not be able to fulfil its function.)
3) *The way a person uses his or her body:* the postures and attitudes adopted; distribution
   of tension and relaxation throughout the body; style of walking and of movement
   generally; special techniques for particular activities (sporting, artistic, etc.); i.e. the
   Use made of it.

People sometimes have difficulty with the concept of *using oneself*. I explain it like this:
suppose I am carrying a heavy tray with both hands. I open the door with my elbow and
switch on the light with my nose. I made a conscious decision to use elbow and nose in
these rather unusual ways. Passing without the tray, I use my hand for both purposes –
so much more obvious a tool that I may well be unaware of having used it. The fact that
I took the use of my hand for granted does not alter the fact that I did use it, as I think
you will agree. Of all our tools, the most immediate are those that are actually part of us.
They are so familiar that we don't always notice our use of them. When F.M. Alexander
called one of his books *The Use of the Self,* some people found the title puzzling. I have
even heard it said that the expression could not be translated into some languages. However, translation became possible as the idea was recognized. Throughout this book, we
shall be looking at ways in which we use ourselves – and at how we think about how we
do this. In this chapter we shall discuss the intimate relation between these three aspects

of the body-image: *Structure, Functioning, and Use.*

When you come to think about it, it is fairly obvious that the way your body functions depends in part on its structure, its very shape. 'Certainly,' you say. 'People with one short leg limp, don't they? People who are all bent over get a crick in the neck just looking where they are going.' Exactly. *Structure affects Functioning.*

We know, too, that the converse is also true: that is, that the way the body functions affects its structure. Muscles that do heavy work become bulkier, affecting the total shape. If an accident causes one leg not to function properly, it sometimes happens that extra strain on the good leg leads to a deterioration in what was previously the good hip-joint. We see that *Functioning affects Structure.*

From common observation, therefore, we can agree that Structure and Functioning affect each other and are interdependent. They affect each other and changes occur in the body. So the body is not quite the fixed entity some people assume it to be. It would be a mistake to think 'I have a body and this is how it is.' Have you ever thought about how the way you use your body affects both its structure and the way it functions? Let us follow the sequence of steps in a deterioration that is, alas, all too common:

1) Imagine that you hold your pen too tightly and get writer's cramp. *(Use affects Functioning.)*
2) If you do it too often, you may lose the inclination to straighten your fingers out again. *(Functioning affects Use.)*
3) If you do it all day every day for years, the day will come when you can no longer straighten them. *(Use affects Structure.)*
4) Because of this, it becomes more difficult to make the up-strokes in your writing. *(Structure affects Functioning.)*
5) In order to form the letters, therefore, you are obliged to increase the movements of bending the fingers and thumb. *(Structure affects Use.)*
6) This in turn increases the cramping effect – and so on...

We can see from this straightforward example that *Use, Structure and Functioning affect each other and are interdependent.* All three aspects are intimately connected and could be viewed schematically like this:

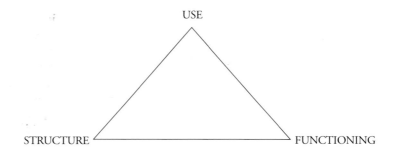

Changes of the kind I have described happen all the time, but because they are gradual we don't always notice them. When we do become aware of the effects, we speak of 'stiffness' or 'old age' – but these are only words, not satisfactory explanations. (I am reminded of the joke about the man who, on being told that the stiffness in his leg was not surprising at his age, replied, 'But, doctor, I have another leg which is perfectly all right, and I've had it just as long as this one.')

Take another common example: by continuous wrong use of the back, we pave the way for the day when a sudden movement or a heavy weight causes a 'slipped disc' or a hernia. We blame the weight or the movement, without understanding that we had already prepared the ground for something to go wrong. We were in fact 'an accident looking for somewhere to happen'. It is nobody's fault, but the fact remains that if we heed only the immediate cause and take no account of the long-term one, we are not being realistic.

It would, however, be a dreadful mistake to suppose that change must necessarily mean deterioration. Well-organized movement, good use of the human organism tends to construct a body whose very shape predisposes it to continued efficiency. We need to modify the old saying 'practice makes perfect'. It is not guaranteed that practice will make perfect – that depends on what has been practised and how, and in what context. But it is highly probable that, for good or ill, whatever we do will take place along lines prepared by repetition. Whether that probability constitutes a threat or a promise depends on how we use ourselves – at all times. Dieticians are fond of telling us 'You are what you eat'. It is at least as true to say 'You are how you move'. Come to that, you are also how you keep still, for both moving and keeping still are ways of using the living body. And, as we have seen, by the way you use it you largely determine its future structure and functioning.

There are people, some of them doctors, who consider that mankind has not – or not yet, anyway – evolved properly for upright posture. They think that this may explain the prevalence of back pain. I do not agree with this view. My work has shown me that even in old age, after a lifetime of misuse, it is frequently possible to restore good functioning – surely an argument for the inherent validity of the design.

I must admit that I sometimes think that such doctors are – understandably – rather too influenced in their thinking by seeing so many sick people all the time! As a teacher, I too see people in whom things have gone wrong; on the other hand, I am fortunate in having the corrective of working with healthy people who want to understand their bodies better in order to achieve even more in their various activities. Each category helps me to understand the other. I sometimes have the pleasure of seeing things that have gone badly wrong, through misuse, go right again once the misuse is corrected. This makes it easier for me to believe that the optimistic view is also the practical one.

Please don't misunderstand me. I am not proposing my sort of teaching as some kind of alternative medicine. I am merely saying that perhaps we misuse the doctor's skills when we ask him or her to 'pick up the pieces' resulting from our mistaken use of ourselves. Poor doctors, they have enough to do treating the sick – no wonder if they sometimes appear pessimistic.

Anyway, let us be practical. Are we to accept the idea of ourselves as an evolutionary dead end, helpless victims of a design fault? Or shall we allow that most of us are the possessors of basically good equipment which we do not always manage to maintain in good working order? Assuming there to be arguments on both sides, which is the more useful hypothesis on which to base our lives?

One thing is sure: we all ought to respect the body enough to use it in accordance with its design. It is not for me to argue about whether that design was created by God or brought about by natural selection – or both. What is clear is that it is not a haphazard muddle. You would not allow an ignorant or clumsy person to fool around with any other complex piece of equipment in your possession. If you would refuse to lend your car to a bad driver, if you have ever forbidden the children to meddle with your sewing machine, you have already realized that *use affects functioning*. Why should it be different with that most wonderful piece of machinery, your own body?

Should you be offended by my referring to your body as machinery, please note that I am not suggesting that it is nothing but a machine. I am just pointing out that there are advantages to understanding and admiring it for the engineering wonder it is.

PART III

ESSENTIAL INFORMATION
(basic)

CHAPTER 6

MUSCLE

People have always eaten people.
What else is there to eat?
If the Ju-ju had meant us not to eat people,
He wouldn't have made us of meat.

Michael Flanders *The Reluctant Cannibal*

Once we start thinking about the Use factor in our body-image, it is fairly obvious that our use of ourselves depends very much on *skeletal muscle:* the means by which we control and move parts of the body in relation to other parts and in relation to our surroundings. (There are other kinds of muscle, dealing with circulation, digestion, etc. I am not going to write about them – for the simple reason that we ourselves cannot do much about these systems, except indirectly by giving them room to function efficiently.)

I have noticed that people are sometimes put off thinking about how they use themselves because they fear that this means, as they put it, 'knowing every muscle and learning to control each one'. They are right to be repelled by this absurd idea. Fortunately nature does not intend us to do anything so complicated. It is true that the *workings* of muscle are very intricate. But from the point of view of a practical handbook such as this, muscle is 'so simple a child can use it'. And of course very young children do use it successfully, without any idea how it works. So much for 'learning to control each muscle'. The only snag really is that if, lurking somewhere in our body-image, there are mistaken ideas about what muscle is and does, then those ideas can cause things to go badly wrong for us – because *thought is reflected in muscle behaviour.*

It is so important to clear away mistaken ideas that I shall risk boring you by spelling out things you know already. In the last thirty years or so I have met many highly intelligent and well-educated people who were nevertheless very ill-informed about muscle, what it is and how it works. Bear with me if I sometimes state what seems to you to be obvious: believe me it is not obvious to everyone. (It ought to be, of course, and it would be if our education had taught us the most necessary facts about ourselves – but how many thinking people would claim unreservedly that our present system of education is a sensible preparation for coping with the realities of life?)

35

I have noticed that when one doesn't know much about a subject, one is often afraid of asking silly questions. Understandable, but regrettable – for the silly questions are the ones it is most important to ask! Here are some I have asked in my time; I shall try to answer them as simply as the facts will allow.

What are muscles, when you come right down to it? I used to find that everyone, from music teachers to journalists writing in beauty magazines, was ready and willing to tell me what to do with my muscles, but nobody made any effort to make sure I knew what they were! Many people suppose, as I once did, that muscles are little strings or pulleys embedded in their flesh. Not so: flesh is muscle. So you see that a lot of your body is muscle: all the meat, in fact (not counting any layers of superfluous fat).

(True story: an anatomy teacher once wanted to show his class what a muscle is like. A vegetarian, he steeled himself to enter a butcher's shop but then realized that he had no idea what to ask for in terms of meat. He tried explaining why he needed 'a muscle' but the butcher said he didn't think they had any! A case of over-specialization on both sides, one might say.)

When you look at meat and see parts of it obviously separated from other parts, that is because the butcher has cut a section across several muscles. Expert carvers know that there is a right and wrong way of carving, according to the grain of the meat – the grain being the muscle fibres. In anatomical drawings, the direction of the muscle fibres is usually shown by many little lines (often red in colour); these lines indicate the direction of pull the particular muscle can exert.

It is a good idea to have a look at some drawings of muscles. Provided you take an all-over view of the body, not forgetting to look at deep muscle layers as well as superficial ones, you will get a useful picture of the multi-directional nature of our muscle-systems. Have a look at figs. 30–34, for example (**Chapter 17**). You need not feel obliged to learn and retain what you see – just looking will help you to efface any over-simplified notions you may have been harbouring unawares – and that will do for the moment.

What is living muscle like? The short answer is: like elastic only more so. By that, I mean that it has something like the pull-back-when-stretched property of elastic, but it can also contract actively, sometimes to shorten its fibres and bunch itself up, sometimes just to prevent itself being stretched. Bear in mind that a muscle can pull or let go but it cannot push. What we know as 'pushing' is a complex activity in which some muscles pull to *stabilize* certain joints, while other joints are opened by the pull exerted by appropriate muscles. This will become clearer as we continue. (**And see Chapter 23: section on Standing up.**)

What happens to muscle when it is in use? We use our muscles by:
1) *Varying their length:* an example occurs when you bend your elbow. This joint is bridged on the inside by muscle attached at one end to bone in your forearm and at the other end to bone in your upper arm. This means that the muscle fibres can contract, shorten themselves and bring the upper arm and forearm nearer to each other, reducing the angle at the elbow joint *(flexion)*. The same kind of thing happens when you increase the angle at the elbow again *(extension)* but in this case the active muscles are those that are attached in such a way that they pass over your elbow on

the outside. The movements known as *flexion* and *extension* are not done by different sorts of muscles; the difference between extensors and flexors lies in where they are attached and hence in the sort of movement they can produce when they contract. (When talking about this sort of thing, it is simplest to use words like *extend, flex, extensor, flexor, extension, flexion*, in their exact sense. These words have precise meaning in anatomy and physiology – this may not always correspond to colloquial use.)

2) *Varying the degree of tension in a muscle:* we do this when we maintain the angle at a joint against resistance (weight or counter-pressure). So we must not jump to the conclusion that contraction always means shortening – nor that relaxation is synonymous with lengthening. Much depends on circumstances, such as the influence of gravity or the opposing action of other muscles. Contraction may actually shorten a muscle, thereby moving a bone. Or it may just cause the muscle to tense enough to maintain its length against resistance – resistance from another muscle or from an outside force, including gravity.

3) *Not varying the length or tension:* it is important to realize that we also use muscles by *not* altering their length or tension. This happens when we maintain them as they are, whether continuing to do the job they are already doing, or just refraining from interfering where they are not wanted.

This last option becomes clearer as we reflect that muscles don't work in isolation. They work in groups (sometimes very large groups running literally from head to toe – and to finger) and their relationships are complex. When you make a movement, any movement, you use:

a) the muscle or muscles responsible for that movement (prime movers);
b) the muscle or muscles which oppose the first set (antagonists) – these have to release, but not too suddenly or the movement would be abrupt;
c) the muscle or muscles which stabilize that part of the body on which the moving part is to move – a gate will not move easily if the gate-post is not firm;
d) the muscle or muscles responsible for maintaining balance of the whole body in the changing situation created by the movement;
e) the muscles responsible for maintaining the shape of the body, the integrity of the structure within or upon which the movement is to occur;
f) you also, consciously or unconsciously, prevent (to some extent, at least) muscle activity which might interfere with what you want to do. This 'negative' use of muscle, is very important and will be explained more fully. (**See Chapter 10.**) You can see that, in fact, **we use the whole system as soon as we use any part of it.**

The same muscle will often play different roles according to circumstances – and sometimes the change of role is very rapid indeed. There are also variations according to whether the movement is gravity-assisted or not. Another point worth noting is that each individual nerve ending controls only some of the fibres of which the muscle is composed. Thus, when a muscle contracts, sometimes only *some* of its fibres join in the activity, and on other occasions they all participate. This arrangement allows of many subtle refinements in our use of muscle.

37

All this is in fact a very simplified description of what occurs when we use our muscles. Even so, you can see now why it would be far too complicated to attempt to control so many interdependent details consciously. Happily for us, our wonderful system of reflexes is capable of making the necessary continuous adaptations, with sufficient speed and accuracy to save us the trouble of calculating and controlling. However, conscious thought can play an important part, by steering the reflex system through the multiplicity of possibilities that present themselves from one split second to the next. We shall discuss this throughout the book, becoming increasingly specific as we proceed. For the moment, what we are asking of conscious thought is to understand the principles involved.

CHAPTER 7

MORE ABOUT MUSCLE

'When I use a word,' Humpty Dumpty said in rather a
scornful tone, 'it means just what I choose it to mean –
neither more or less.'

'The question is,' said Alice, 'whether you can make
words mean so many different things.'

Lewis Carroll *Through the Looking-Glass*

It will be obvious to the reader that, even using everyday language and the absolute
minimum of technical vocabulary, we shall sometimes need to pause to define terms –
for very practical reasons. This seems to be a moment when such definition is needed, if
we are to understand each other clearly. Somewhere, in the midst of the confusion
that for most of us constitutes what ought to be a clear body-image, are to be found such
words and expressions as *relaxation, tension, stretching, muscle slackness, strength,
weakness, toning up, etc.* – terms which attempt to describe muscular behaviour, while
not being completely clear to many of the people who bandy them about. In this chapter, we shall try to discuss their meaning in the light of what is known about the nature
and properties of muscle.

Relaxation (In this context, *to relax = make or become loose or slack* – according to the
Oxford English Dictionary.)

We are here dealing with what is probably one of the most misused words in the
language. Nowadays, people who are aware of being what they call 'tense' are apt to talk
as if *tension* were bad and *relaxation* good. This is nonsense – and dangerous nonsense at
that. We need both, properly distributed, all the time, as long as we live, even when we
are asleep.

As you can understand from the previous chapter, the distribution of tension and relaxation is constantly changing and very complex – much too complex, in fact, to be
dealt with by direct interference, as we shall see. Loose talk about 'moving in a relaxed
way' does not help anyone – it only encourages muddled thinking and hence, muddled
action. Let us forget for a moment all the (perhaps useful) things that this expression
may have stood for to some people at some time. Instead, let's examine it logically. By relaxing, you can drop some part of you that you have previously lifted; you can drop an

39

object by ceasing to hold it; or you can fall to the ground. You will agree that this leaves many of our movements unaccounted for! The rest of our actions are accomplished by muscular contraction, by muscles pulling on bones, thereby causing them to move in relation to other bones. So 'moving in a relaxed way' is a meaningless expression.

Even sillier, when you come to think about it, is the often heard 'he is so completely relaxed' – referring to someone carrying out a skilled task. One hears this over and over again during television showing of tennis tournaments, for instance. The only reasonable answer is 'No, he isn't. If he were as relaxed as it is possible to be, he would be lying on the floor in a heap. And even then his breathing muscles would be working.' *Nature does not permit complete relaxation* – luckily for us.

I think we should all try to defend language from these assaults, otherwise the day will come when we can no longer use words to communicate usefully with each other. Granted that some things are not easy to express, we could still take a little more trouble with our words. (Humpty Dumpty at least paid the words extra when he asked them to mean something they *don't* mean.) I insist on this point because this kind of talk has led countless people into serious physical difficulties, by giving them the idea that they can somehow accomplish something by making themselves go all floppy. The result is usually that they relax what they *can* relax, without any guarantee that this is what *should* be relaxed. The upshot of such meddling is, very often, extra work for muscles that are already overworking. The outcome can be misery untold.

An aspect of the problem is that what *feels* like relaxation may really be the *giving way*, by one set of muscles, to a continuous strong pull from an opposing muscle group. For example, I often find that people who look very collapsed have certain abdominal muscles that are disproportionately strong. They stop fighting the pulling-down effect of these muscles, call it 'relaxing' – and frequently end up with back trouble. Direct attempts to 'strengthen the back' are not a solution. (See the paragraph below on *Strength and weakness*.) It is all too easy to fall into this trap, which is very dangerous, because the whole framework of the body depends on a delicate balance and co-operation between opposing muscle groups.

So far we have been talking about the kind of 'relaxation' that takes place, or that we can induce, as we go about our normal activities. Now I should like to mention an even more serious risk. I have occasionally come across people who had practised conscious relaxation to such a point that they could render themselves heavy, slack, and virtually unprepared for any kind of movement whatsoever. This, fortunately, is rare, for it takes a lot of practice! It is hard to see what good it can do anyone. Some people claim it helps them to sleep, but scientists tell us that a lot of movement takes place during healthy sleep. A dog or cat asleep feels peaceful but lively to the touch – quite different from the collapsed state that confused human thinking often supposes desirable. In the words of the athletics coach Percy Cerutty:

> where the science and art of delivering full power without stress and strain is understood, the word 'relaxation' is seldom used.[1]

Muscular efficiency

We have seen that it is misleading to speak of 'relaxation' when marvelling at the economy of effort shown by a skilled person performing a complicated task. What we are in fact admiring is an appropriateness of performance, a readiness of response to the owner's intentions, on the part of muscles maintained in a constantly-adapting working balance. This is easier to understand when we note that one of the properties of muscle is that *the most effective contraction is made when the muscle concerned is already slightly stretched to begin with.*

To make this clearer: a muscle that is being slightly stretched is, by its nature, already slightly pulling against the stretch, i.e. it is beginning to pull in the direction of its contraction. In this respect it is like elastic. (**See Chapter 6, and the paragraph on Stretch, below.**) This slight stretch, and the muscle's reflex reaction to being stretched, take up the slack in the muscle, making it lively and ready for work. Then, every bit of contraction it can do within itself becomes effective (assuming it is the right muscle for the job in hand). But, just as the elastic in your waistband, if not subjected to a bit of stretch, could not be expected to accomplish much, so it is difficult for a very slack muscle to contract itself enough to be ready to achieve anything.

Excessive contraction

Excessive contraction is also an obstacle to efficiency. There is, of course, a limit to how much contraction a muscle can achieve, so naturally, if it is over-contracted before starting the work you want it to do, it hasn't got much scope for doing more, however willing it is to carry out your wishes. Moreover, when you want to make a movement in the opposite direction, too much work will be demanded of the opposing muscle. In quick repeated movements, this sort of escalating battle between opposing muscles does not allow either muscle the time needed to lengthen out between contractions. It is very tiring and can bring the movement to a standstill quite quickly. So much work and no result! Athletes in Victorian times called this being *muscle-bound* – an expression which seems to have fallen into disuse but which is nevertheless very descriptive. I have seen violinists come to this within a few minutes, with certain quick repeated bowing movements. In the long term, you can do the same sort of thing to yourself, if you habitually contract your muscles for no useful purpose, squashing in on yourself instead of maintaining an expanded framework within which muscles have room to work properly.

All this explains why *neither slack muscles nor over-contracted ones are efficient.* Muscles have a fair chance of doing their job properly only when they can depend on the skeletal framework being maintained in a balanced state of expansion. When I speak of muscles working 'properly', I mean that the result you want is obtained with the *minimum effort appropriate to the task;* that is what muscular efficiency is. Sometimes minimum effort may be quite a lot of effort! That is fine, if the effort is appropriate and applied correctly.

❑ *Experiment* (for those who know how to play cat's cradle)

Take about 150 cm. of narrow elastic and join up the ends. Get someone to play cat's cradle with you. You will understand quite a lot about the necessity of maintaining a slight stretch, for you will see how things become disorganized if you don't. You can also discover what happens if the elastic is pulled very tight. I sometimes get my students to play cat's cradle – it is quite surprising how much easier it is to discuss this kind of thing with them afterwards. (If you don't know cat's cradle, ask your grandmother.)

Strength and weakness

In practical terms, the moral of all this is: if some of your muscles appear to be 'weak', they may in fact merely have reached the limit of their capacity for work. Perhaps they are already working inappropriately hard, doing just about all they can, or ever *should* do. In that case, they will not respond to so-called 'strengthening exercises'. The question is, not how to strengthen them, but how to render their effort effective. They may be working too hard because of conditions elsewhere: perhaps other muscles are pulling against them, as described above; or possibly, elsewhere in the system, some muscles ought to be joining in, but are not doing their share of the work. *There can be several reasons for apparent weakness.* So be warned against jumping to conclusions. (See also Chapter 19.)

Stretch

You might think that the answer to over-contraction would be to stretch the muscles out again. But stretching exercises are not the automatic answer to this problem, because of another property of muscle, known as the *stretch reflex*. This is the characteristic tendency of muscle, when stretched, to pull back to where it came from (like elastic).

We most often think of muscles as things that move us around, and this is true. But they are also things that keep us from falling apart: a function which they share with various kinds of connective tissue. Their 'primary function ... is the "relationing" of the various parts of the body to one another...'[2] and 'to respond to disconnection by resisting it ... Muscles in their very nature are built to be sensitive to stretch and to respond by resisting that stretch...'[3] F.P. Jones wrote:

> One stimulus to which a muscle responds by contracting is mechanical stretch. Stretch can be applied by an outside force like gravity or an inside force like the hydraulic pressure in the disks or by the contraction of other muscles. The tension generated in a muscle is proportional to the stretching force, but it can be modified ... by mechanisms in the nervous system that respond both to feedback from the muscle ... and to signals from other parts of the organism.[4]

Jones also quotes Sherrington, describing posture as a 'congeries of stretch reflexes'.[5] Stretch reflexes are enormously important: they are operative, not only in *what we do*, but also in *how we are*. Besides providing a measure of safeguard against overreaching our capacities, they operate with great subtlety and discrimination: it seems that the feedback system mentioned by Jones – which Gorman considers 'actually a more complex error-activated feedforward system'[6] – is capable of comparing our intentions and the actual conditions in our muscles.

One should always hesitate to interfere with such a delicate mechanism. If you think some of your muscles are too contracted, my advice is, *don't make efforts to stretch them. You may very well stimulate them to contract more.* At worst, you may damage them, for it can happen that the active part of a muscle is willing to stretch but is being restricted by connective tissue. An ounce of caution is worth a ton of well-meant exercises. What then can you do about it? Patience! Consideration of basic information is a necessary procedure if positive steps described later are to be effective.

(The workings of the stretch reflex may also present an argument for avoiding treatment by 'traction' unless it is absolutely necessary to avoid nerve damage or to bring together displaced parts which must heal and knit together, e.g. after an accident. If traction is offered to you as a treatment for 'backache', I do suggest you ask your doctor if there is anything less drastic that could be tried first – or perhaps even seek a second opinion. I am not a doctor and I hate to appear critical of them, for I realize, gratefully, that they know many valuable things that I don't know. But, in all modesty, I cannot help recognizing that, as a teacher of movement and co-ordination, I have acquired a certain amount of specialized knowledge that is not included in medical training. In the light of experience, I feel obliged to say that, having seen a number of people who have previously had treatment by traction, so far I have only come across one person who claimed to be 'right as rain' afterwards. The others seemed to have been both frightened and weakened by it, and I would say that their general co-ordination appeared to be suffering. I was aware of a lack of elasticity in them, a missing confidence in movement. I can, of course, appreciate how necessary it seemed at the time to find some, *any* relief from pain.

The real answer is never to let things get to that state. It is *not* self-indulgent to make the time to find out how to correct your mistakes before they do serious damage – but too many people leave it far too late and then expect the doctor to wave a magic wand over them, so that they can continue to inflict ill-treatment on their own long-suffering body.)

Slack muscles

As I mentioned earlier, sometimes a muscle is not ready to work because it is too slack. An example can be found in the abdominal musculature. These muscles, when they really co-operate properly with one another and with the rest of the body, act like a sort of ideally designed elastic corset to keep things comfortably in place without restricting our freedom. (See figs. 33, 34, Chapter 17.) But if one muscle is too contracted, another may well be slack as a result. Here, logically, stretching exercises might seem to be the answer – but beware! You cannot always be sure *which* muscle you are stretching. It may be that the over-contraction of some muscles, as described above, is the real cause of slackness in others: by interfering with the shape of the bony framework, it has robbed other muscles of the opportunity to start work from a stretched state. It is hard to imagine a stretching exercise that could remedy the situation.

All in all, in ordinary life, specific exercises are rarely the solution to such problems and are better avoided. Even where special preparatory exercises have been designed for special techniques of dance, athletics, music, etc., it is important always to establish the true, easy balance between the muscle groups of the whole body, before embarking on such specialized training. A wise coach will always take this into account.

Where does this leave us? Well, take heart! Some different approaches, apparently more indirect, are none the less effective. The more we progress with putting together the jigsaw of our body-image, the better you will see how these approaches can work.

To explain in detail how muscle works would be very complicated and outside the scope of this book. I have tried here to single out those aspects where a better understanding can be of practical use in daily life. The whole purpose is to help you to base your body-image on facts.

To sum up, we may say that there are essentially two types of muscular inadequacy: slackness and over-contraction. Their interaction is complicated, which is why a direct attack on either is seldom successful. The only true solution is to establish a gently expanding framework for the activity of the entire musculature. We shall start to discuss this in the next chapter.

Information about the workings of muscle can be found in Gray's *Anatomy* (Myology section). Other sources referred to in the text:

1. Percy Wells Cerutty, *Athletics – how to become a champion*, London, Stanley Paul, 1960.
2. R.A. Dart, 'Voluntary musculature in the human body: the double-spiral arrangement', *British Journal of Physical Medicine*, 1950, reprinted in Dart, *Skill and Poise*, London, STAT Books, 1996, p. 59.
3. David Gorman, 'In our own image', *Alexander Review*, 1987, vol. 2, no. 1. Reprinted in D. Gorman, *Looking at Ourselves*, Learning Methods, 1997, pp. 33–9.
4. F.P. Jones, *Freedom to Change*, London, Mouritz, 1997, p. 142.
5. *ibid.* p. 144.
6. Gorman, *op. cit.*

CHAPTER 8

MUSCLES AND THE FRAMEWORK

It is better to do nothing than to do harm. Half the useful work in the world consists of combating the harmful work. A little time spent in learning to appreciate facts is not time wasted, and the work that will be done afterwards is far less likely to be harmful...

Bertrand Russell *The Conquest of Happiness*

So far, we have talked about muscles and the ways in which they influence each other. This influence is exerted chiefly via the bones on which the muscles act. For it is the function of muscles to act on bones, either by moving them or by maintaining the relationship of one bone to another. How do the various bits of us behave in relation to each other? The question is unavoidable, since, as we have seen, the whole is involved in any use of the parts.

Sooner or later, in this sort of discussion, someone is bound to come up with the dreaded word *posture*. This is a word I don't much care for, perhaps because it so often has the words *good* or *bad* attached to it. Preceded by *good*, it conjures up pictures of soldiers standing to attention, of Victorian young ladies balancing books on their heads. It sounds rigid. When *bad* is the adjective associated with it, feelings of guilt and rebellion can be aroused – and both of these emotions carry us further from good use of ourselves.

Let me give you an example. In my private teaching I have often had to deal with people who were what is commonly called 'round-shouldered'. If one knows what one is doing, it is usually fairly easy to help them. The people who are much harder to help are those who *feel* like letting their shoulders drop forward, but who believe that they *ought* to keep them back, that 'good posture' requires them to 'make the effort'. However, keeping their shoulders back makes them feel 'tense', so then they think that they *ought* to 'relax'. As we have seen (**in Chapter 7**) they probably have no idea of *what* to relax.

By the time these people have fiddled about with all the permutations, without any clear view of what the choices really are, the whole situation has become more than a little complicated. I met a woman of about sixty who had been in this double bind since childhood, when ill-informed advice *(sit up straight! shoulders back!)* had set her off on a lifetime of discomfort. Worse, she had always had feelings of inadequacy, associated with her inability to do as she was told. She wept with relief when I showed her that her parents, with the best of intentions, had made a fundamental mistake when they instilled that first *'ought'*. (**See Chapter 24.**)

Not everyone tries so hard to obey parental advice to pull the shoulders back. There are those who get fed up with the whole thing, and express rebellion by slumping aggressively; this is supposed to show how 'relaxed', how 'cool' they are – but it can often be recognized as an attempt at masking problems. Again, there are the people who, when seated, alternate between a) a slump that does nobody any good, and b) what they think of as 'good posture' or 'sitting up straight'. A more accurate description of b) might be 'tilting your pelvis and hollowing your back, to hide – even from yourself – the fact that you are really still slumping'. This alternation is very tiring and its consequences are unpleasant. I ought to know: I did it for years and it did me a great deal of harm!

I saw a good example of this pointless correcting and re-correcting (into which we can all fall so easily) in a retired regimental sergeant-major who told me that his back had begun to hurt. Until then, I had known him as an exceptionally happy person. Since his early retirement he was doing a job he particularly liked; he was good at it, and was living in the place of his dreams. The work, however, was physically demanding, and the pain in his back began to threaten not only his health but his livelihood and his home. Everything he most enjoyed in life was suddenly at risk. When we discussed the problem, he was quick to recognize that for most of his adult life he had been alternating between two contrasting ways of carrying himself: one was the rigid military bearing required by the army, the other was an off-duty slump that he thought of as restful. Fortunately, his physique was fundamentally good, and he had a natural preference for the happy medium once it had been explained to him – but I rage at the thought of lives that have been ruined unnecessarily by this sort of thing.

So I shall try to avoid the word *posture*. In view of all its associations, it seems unlikely to help our discussion much. However, we do need a word to indicate the relationship between the various bits of us. The old-fashioned word *carriage* has the double advantage of suggesting movement and of implying that weight and substance have to be coped with. *Framework* is another useful word. I have used it already, and now I should like to examine its implications in more detail.

The framework I mean consists, broadly speaking, of bones and muscles. It is a two-purpose structure which provides a protective casing for the organs that are our life-support system, enclosing them within a sort of reinforced tube, while at the same time supplying the means of transporting this casing and its precious contents from place to place. Whether going about or staying in one spot, it can balance itself in various attitudes and extend bits of itself to interact with the world around us. This moveable framework thus gives us both protection and adaptability. Within and around it, we can make an infinite variety of movements. But much will depend on the way it is used and managed.

The last two chapters dealt mainly with muscles. What should we bear in mind about the role of *bones* in the framework? Gray's says:

> Bone tissue and the skeletal struts and levers formed of it, are evidently adapted with exquisite precision to resist all forms of stress, and with a suitable degree of resilience, in the varying play of musculature. The skeleton is sometimes said to give shape to the body: but the shape itself is largely an expression of the characteristic motor activities...[1]

The last sentence quoted refers to the shape of different animal species being determined by the movements the animal typically performs. It is also fair to say that the shape of different *individual* humans is largely an expression of the muscle activity characteristic of each person.

We shall do well to reflect on the qualities of bone tissue, which Gray's summarizes thus:

> Bone is essentially a highly vascular, living, constantly changing, mineralized connective tissue ... remarkable for its hardness, resilience, characteristic growth mechanisms and its regenerative capacity.[2]

People tend to forget that bone is 'living, constantly changing'. We all know that broken bones do mend; that apart, I find many people reluctant to believe that anything about their skeleton can ever improve. This seems illogical, in view of their readiness to accept deterioration. It is worth remembering that the skeleton, too, is a living part of our framework. It, too, is inevitably *used* – or sometimes misused – by the owner.

In this connection, I remember with pleasure a little girl whose doctor sent her to me with a scoliosis, a condition which is often described in text-books as a lateral curvature of the spine; Carrington points out that it is in fact 'a corkscrew-like condition'[3]. The doctor wanted, if possible, to avoid orthopaedic treatment for this child and asked me to see what I could do. Faced with a lively six-year-old, keen on her violin lessons and her dancing class, it was not easy to explain why I wanted her temporarily to set aside these activities. Fortunately, she was extremely bright and could understand the importance of learning to do things without associated harmful habits coming into play. She co-operated fully and it was a happy day, some months later, when the doctor said, 'Well, she certainly did have a scoliosis – and she certainly hasn't got one now'.

That experience taught me that Alexander's message can be got across in more ways than one: the friendliness of this child, in the many hours we spent together each weekend, afforded opportunities for all sorts of work and play. There was no planned structure; things were mostly pretty casual but always turned around the theme of 'doing *this* without doing *that*', accompanied by very slight tactile indications on my part. Muscle is instantly responsive to our slightest thought; changes in bony structures take place much more slowly – and when they do, it is often in response to changes in muscle behaviour. Nothing stands still, and change can be for better or for worse. *It quite often happens that good changes establish themselves simply because we stop provoking bad changes.*

Bone is a specialized form of connective tissue. The basic material known as *connective tissue* assumes different forms and textures to suit the site and function of the different components of the framework. These forms include:

a) *Cartilage* (gristle) The framework includes several types of cartilage, providing elasticity and protecting bone from friction, especially at joint surfaces.[4]

b) *Ligaments* Occurring at joints, these are tough cords or bands, holding bones together. Despite their strength, they are flexible and offer no resistance to normal movements, being designed to prevent excessive or abnormal movements.[5] Jones points out that ligaments 'can only function at their normal length'.[6] Thus it is only by balanced use of our muscles that we can ensure that the ligaments have the chance to save us from ourselves.

c) *Tendons* Tough cords or straps joining muscle to bone. Each muscle fibre has a tiny sheath of fine connective tissue to which muscle is attached – each bundle of muscle fibres also has a sheath of connective tissue and so does the whole muscle. All these sheaths run the length of the muscle to join up at the ends, forming tendons.[7]

d) *Aponeuroses* Broad sheets of dense connective tissue to which muscle is attached – not all muscles being attached directly to bone.[8]

e) *Fascia* A wide term which 'signifies little more than a collection of connective tissue large enough to be described by the unaided eye'.[9] Such connective tissue is significant for the framework where it occurs between muscles which move extensively on each other, presumably to facilitate movement. (In some places the deep fascia resembles an aponeurosis and performs the same function.)

Ideally, the ensemble of the bones keeps the muscles just slightly stretched and thus ready to work efficiently when called upon (see **Chapter** 7) and the muscles keep the bones in place. It is rather like the relationship between the frame and the strings of a tennis racquet: the frame keeps the strings taut enough, and the strings prevent warping of the frame. Of course, it is much more complicated than that, because the set-up of a tennis racquet, though it has to be able to cope with the stresses of impact, does not have to allow for maintaining the integrity of its essential structure while actively bending and twisting itself.

Without bone, the body would be just a floppy mass, about as much use to us as a tent with no tent-pole. Without muscle, the bones would lie in a heap on the floor; the spinal column itself, bereft of its muscles, tendons, ligaments, cartilage, instead of being the main upright support, would resemble a collection of oddly-shaped beads, incapable of supporting itself, let alone anything else.

Some of our muscles are chiefly concerned with preventing distortion of the framework. Some are more occupied in interacting with the environment by moving the framework about in space, or parts of it in relation to other parts. Some have a double role to play. Many are involved in the moment-by-moment business of keeping us balanced in the vertical. To understand how the framework can be maintained or distorted, let us take a look at major muscle-systems. A detailed study of individual muscles could get too complex for our purposes. The important practical point here is that *muscles do not work in isolation: each one acts within a constantly adapting framework, influencing and being influenced by other muscles.* (**Chapter** 6)

It is valid to describe muscles as organizing themselves into large head-to-toe systems, each of which tends to act as a group in relation to other muscle-systems. By studying these groups, we can get a useful idea of the organization of the musculature as a whole and how it determines our basic shape and attitudes.[10,11]

When we are in the womb, we are folded up, and the shape of the spinal column follows a curve, known as the primary curve. Once born, we can and do arch also in the opposite direction. The primary curve is not lost, but, as we grow up, secondary curves in this opposite direction start to appear in the spinal column: in the neck and the small of the back. In the course of our early attempts at moving ourselves, we discover that we have muscles for making ourselves either shape: there is a muscle-system in front for curling ourselves up, and another behind for arching backwards. Later, the ability to stand upright will depend on our somehow achieving a balance of pulls between these two muscle-systems, and thus a balance of primary and secondary curves.

Looking at it mechanically, you will understand that imbalance means that, rather than fall down, the person resorts to all sorts of complicated muscular compensations which make life more tiring and difficult. So the balance between primary and secondary curves is intimately concerned in the efficiency or otherwise of the balancing act we all perform throughout our waking hours. Moreover, too little curve, or too much, will result in inefficient placing of weight and stress – and hence, eventually, in damage to the structure, and in reduction of the springy quality of its support.

You can readily see that, in standing, if one of these muscle-systems is too slack, the least activity of the other can unbalance the whole structure. You can see, too, that if one system is pulling too hard, the other will have to work extra hard to compensate. It is rather like putting up a tent: if the tent is leaning to one side, we have to decide whether your ropes need tightening or those on my side need slackening off. Furthermore, if one system works too hard, the opposing system, in compensating, pulls against it, thus stimulating it to work even harder! (Chapter 7, stretch reflex) The second, in turn, reacts against this, and so on, until, instead of co-operation between the two systems, we have *something like an escalating war*. As in war, it is not easy for either side to reduce its forces, because of the risks involved in an imbalance of power.

However, if the imbalance is allowed to continue, the whole structure will become distorted, cramped, weakened. To continue the tent analogy, if we both keep on tightening our ropes, and if the ropes don't give way or dislodge the tent-pegs, the pole will break or be driven into the ground. In the human body, besides damage to the spinal column, one thing that suffers in a conflict between front and back is a third muscle-system, linking front and back: a system of somewhat trampoline-like muscles, including the pelvic floor, diaphragm, soft palate, and the arches of the feet. In an escalating war (or even cold war) between front and back, these muscles, which contribute to a delicate system of interior springing, lose some of their springy nature – with disastrous consequences, for we then bear down on ourselves, creating stresses that neither joints nor internal organs were ever meant to stand up to.

These three systems share a good deal of the responsibility for holding us up, but our musculature does not stop at these three. We also have muscle-systems concerned with twisting movements of the trunk and with movements of the arms and legs. Again, some of these movements are of the kind where we fold in on ourselves at the front of the body; others are more of the sideways and backwards variety. Again, both are necessary and neither should dominate. Again, there is danger of escalation, if our efforts to correct a dominant tendency are pursued with too much enthusiasm.

When major muscle groups cease to be locked in an escalating war, when instead they start to co-operate, one can begin to appreciate the way they wrap us around in a 'broad, torso-encompassing' double spiral, as described by Dart.[12] How do different muscles, even different muscle layers, relate and co-operate? If this is not immediately obvious to you when you consider the trunk, you can certainly get an idea by thinking about the musculature of the limbs, for it would clearly be a mistake to suppose that arm muscles are only in the arms, or leg muscles only in the legs.

❏ *Experiment*:

Rest the whole of your forearm on the table and drum with your fingers: you will see muscles at work in your forearm although the arm itself is not moving. Similarly, muscles can be seen at work in the upper arm when the forearm moves – the biceps is an obvious example. In fact the muscle-system of the upper limb can be traced all the way from the 'business end' (the tips of your fingers and thumb) to the small of your back, as well as across the shoulders to the spine at the same level, across the front to the breast-bone, and by several routes all the way up to your head. This means that conditions in the back affect the efficiency of your fingers and vice versa.

Similarly, muscles responsible for leg movements are also to be found attached to the lumbar spine (small of the back) and a similar two-way influence holds good. Do you begin to see, therefore, how the arms and legs influence each other, how the whole system links up? We shall also see how the attitude of the head exerts a very significant influence on everything. (**Chapters 13–17**) First, however, we shall look at some of the ways in which thoughts and feelings can influence muscle use – and vice versa.

---

1. Gray's *Anatomy*, Longman, Edinburgh, 1973, 35th edition, p. 206 (Osteology).
2. *ibid.* p. 215.
3. W. Carrington and S. Carey, *Explaining the Alexander Technique*, London, Sheildrake, 1992, p. 135.
4. Gray's *Anatomy*, p. 210 (Osteology).
5. *ibid.* p. 395 (Arthrology).
6. F.P. Jones, *Freedom to Change*, London, Mouritz, 1997, p. 143.
7. Gray's *Anatomy*, p. 488 (Myology).
8. *ibid.* p. 489.
9. *ibid.* p. 490.
10. R.A. Dart, 'Voluntary musculature in the human body: the double-spiral arrangement', *British Journal of Physical Medicine*, (1950) reprinted in Dart, *Skill and Poise*, London, STAT Books, 1996.
11. G. Struyf-Denys, *Les Chaînes musculaires et articulaires,* Société Belge d'Ostéopathie et de Recherche en Thérapie Manuelle, 1978.
12. R.A. Dart, *op. cit.* p. 69.

CHAPTER 9

MUSCLES AND MOOD

... speces of thynges and progressiouns
Shullen enduren by successiouns,
And nat eterne, withouten any lye.
This maystow understonde and seen at ye.

Chaucer *The Canterbury Tales: The Knight's Tale*

(Things of all kinds, all processes, survive
By continual succession, do not live
For ever and ever. And this is no lie,
As anyone can see with half an eye.
Translation by David Wright)

The muscle-systems we have just been discussing, these head-to-toe organizations of muscle which determine our shape and physical attitudes, are closely associated with our moods and even with more enduring personal characteristics. Our very language reflects this fact. We speak of someone *looking as if he had the weight of the world on his shoulders.* We say *my back is broad* – meaning *I can cope, I can take it.* Circumstances may *get us down*; friends or opportunities are welcomed *with open arms.* There is the *outgoing* type of person and the *drooping flower.* I may be *in an expansive mood*, or *just keeping my head above water.* Somebody might express shame or embarrassment by saying *I just don't know how I shall ever hold my head up again.* Faced with an unpleasant task one *just grits one's teeth and gets on with it.* And so on.

What this kind of language so vividly expresses is the unity of the individual human being. The intuitive wisdom of everyday speech recognizes no mind-body split. If I am depressed or if I feel great, it is *I* who feel depressed or great, not my body or my mind. There is a coherence, a consistency, between 'inner' and 'outer' states – and that is fine, so far as it goes. There is indeed a time for curling up and getting cosy, a time for a bracing, stimulating walk in the wind, a time for reticence and a time for being 'outgoing', a time for concentration and a time for a more 'wide-angled' state of observation; a time for grief, for anger, for jumping for joy; for determination, for calm acceptance: and each of these states of being of the whole person has naturally its typical attitudes and muscular conditions.

All this is normal, essential even; and it is also fine that some people by nature tend more one way or the other. What is *not* fine is when people become so fixed in one of

51

these attitudes that they cannot adopt another, even one that would be more appropriate, more in accordance with their real wishes.

Imagine, for instance, a girl in her early twenties, who has been quite shy during her growing years – perhaps self-conscious about her height or her developing figure – and so has adopted what at first was no more than a *habit* of hanging her head and hugging her arms. Add to this that she is very fond of her much younger sister, and has spent a good deal of time cuddling the child and stooping protectively over her. On top of this, she is academically gifted and has spent long hours at her desk, expressing concentration by turning, not only her gaze, but her neck and shoulders too, down and inwards towards the work in front of her. She has always felt at ease and happy with her little sister and in her studies, so she quite likes her stooping attitude; she feels at home in it. Nevertheless, if she had been less shy, she would naturally have emerged from it when walking, dancing, chatting with contemporaries. In fact, for a long time, it was only shyness that prevented her coming out of her habitual 'round-shouldered' stoop – but with time the muscles have settled for the length that feels familiar, the bones have got pulled into a more or less stable relationship to one another.

One day she has to go for a job interview. The job in question would suit her capabilities. Obviously it is important to her to let the interviewer see this by her answers – she's not too worried about that. But, things being what they are, she knows that it is also important to be able to look confident and to have an air of being easy to get along with. She looks at herself in the mirror, trying to judge the effect she will have – and finds that she doesn't in fact *look* very confident. She isn't even sure, come to think of it, that her clothes are hanging as they should. Observing herself, she starts to feel less sure of herself than she did before. She tries different stances but nothing seems to make a lot of difference. She is only young but she has already spent too long allowing physical expression to only some aspects of her character – and now she seems likely to be stuck with the 'personality' to which she has given bodily form.

If only this had occurred to her sooner, she could have used the moments when she wasn't feeling particularly shy, protective, or concentrated – and taken the opportunity to let her body bounce back into shape, as it were. It is not too late to reverse the process, but unless she gets expert help, it may now be difficult for her to attempt this without provoking the escalation effect. **(Chapter 8)**

It would be easier to understand – and therefore to avoid – what has happened, if we could look at a speeded-up version of such changes occurring – like those films of flowers growing. In fact, a speeded-up effect can sometimes be observed in athletes, particularly in endurance events. I once saw a world-class athlete reach such a state of fatigue that the muscles supporting the spine were no longer strong enough to resist a personal tendency to curl up in front. This tendency, normally slight, was at the time grossly exaggerated by the demands being placed on the whole organism. The imbalance of pulls on the entire structure of the body became such that it was equally impossible to continue or to stop – the only possible result was to fall. Verticality, which had depended on what we have called *escalation*, was no longer possible when it became simply too tiring to maintain the escalation.

I feel one should be grateful to athletes who have the courage to expose themselves to such ordeals. The value for the rest of us lies in the chance to understand, in a short space of time, a process that in normal circumstances would take much longer to develop visible results. What I saw in this case, in the course of a few hours, could teach us something about what the passage of years can do to people who habitually achieve results by escalating means: that is, we could learn something about what is often (thoughtlessly) referred to as 'the ageing process'. Since not all elderly people develop a stoop and associated inconveniences, the use of the word *ageing* in this context makes highly undesirable assumptions about what we should and should not accept as normal.

(There was a woman to whom I gave Alexander lessons many years ago: she was then in her sixties, a biologist. Now and then I would receive from her delightful and challenging letters, some of which I still have. In one that I treasure particularly, she wrote:

> Daily walk to station took me 35 minutes ... now 22 minutes and no breathlessness...; why should I *know* that to attempt to *run* ... at my age would *be* foolish – not just *look* foolish? *What is senescence?*

And in another, after describing health improvements and a renewed zest for intellectual work, she added:

> One *dis*advantage – I had come to terms with Death – genuinely, and suitably at my age; this is no longer so; life is beckoning hard...

As I grow older myself, I think of those letters when I am tempted to think that this or that difficulty belongs to my age.)

It is normal to want to give appropriate physical expression to feelings and states of mind – indeed, not to do so can in some cases feel like some kind of lie or betrayal of oneself. Most people at some time have to cope with bereavements, shocks, disappointments: fortunate are those who can allow themselves space both to live these experiences *and* to move on from them. Many people also encounter high points of excitement: fortunate are those who can live them joyfully – and still handle the humdrum moments. As far as our reactions are concerned, the real issue is one of degree and duration. There is a natural wish, even a need, to use the body to express emotions, moods, personality traits – even if at times this means departing from the 'happy medium'. There is also a need to retain the possibility of an expanded, balanced framework. Between these two needs we have to maintain a balance, lest we become what popular wisdom calls *unbalanced!*

Remember that (here too, as with the more mechanical kind of balance we were discussing in the last chapter) the way to improved balance is not to be found by escalation, by forcing yourself against your natural inclination. It can be found by reminding yourself that you actually possess sets of characteristics other than your dominant ones – albeit in different proportions. Realize that it is not necessary to push yourself two hundred per cent into any attitude or state of being. However whole-hearted you are in what you are doing or in what you are feeling, there must come a moment when you are free to move in another direction, if only temporarily. I can assure you that the simple awareness of this fact, combined with consciously allowing it to be so on a mundane muscular level, has helped many people to cope with circumstances that were difficult on a level usually thought of as 'psychological'. If you want to put this to the test, it is usually best,

53

as in other skills, to practise on something easy, so here are a couple of experiments you may like to make.

❑ *Experiment 1*

When you are carrying something heavy, remember that your hands are also capable of opening out and letting go of what they are holding. This thought lessens the likelihood of holding the object more tightly than necessary. As a result, your hands will probably release their grip more easily when the appropriate moment comes for setting down the load.

❑ *Experiment 2*

When keeping still, just admit the possibility of turning your head or moving a limb – remembering that these movements are available to you, even if you do not choose to make them just now.

By such experiments, you will be laying for yourself the foundations of a balanced structure that will not topple too far in any one direction. Which of us can tell when the moment will come when we need all the resilience we can muster? Experience in the kind of thinking described above, in situations as banal as those I have just mentioned, can be of inestimable value in coping with life's major upsets. I have seen people use this approach in recovering from serious illness, from emotional tragedy, from all sorts of set-backs. Nevertheless, I should not presume to recommend it to you if I were not also speaking from personal experience.

CHAPTER 10

MUSCLES AND CHOICE

The most important factor is ... the power not to respond in the usual way ...
Its absence would negate the very possibility of adaptive variability in behaviour.
David Stenhouse *The Evolution of Intelligence*

At least we have the power to choose what we will not do.
Walter Carrington

Throughout this book, it is suggested that some of the movements that are available to us might be better avoided, or performed less often, or accomplished by means other than those we take for granted. This of course implies that choices are open to us, as indeed they are, to a far greater extent than people often suppose. All day long, in all our movements, every little component of each action has superseded a multitude of other possibilities: has in fact been *chosen*, consciously or not. Obviously, much more is involved than the framework and its controlling musculature. Many levels of the brain and nervous system are concerned in the slightest gesture. Gray's *Anatomy* says of the human nervous system that 'its structure and activities are inseparably interwoven with every aspect of our lives, physical, cultural and intellectual.'[1]

One aspect of all this activity deserves our particular attention. The great neurologist Sir Charles Sherrington emphasized that:

> ... to refrain from an act is no less an act than to commit one, because inhibition is co-equally with excitation a nervous activity.[2]

Nervous activity of course means in this context 'activity of the nervous system'. *Inhibition* (Sherrington used the word in its technical sense) is the partner and opposite of *excitation*; it is the non-activation of mechanisms. F.M. Alexander used 'inhibition' to mean non-activation of mechanisms *when their action would be inappropriate to a desired end*. (Chapter 34) For an understanding of the work of these two men, it is important to know that, in their vocabulary, inhibition has nothing to do with the colloquial sense of suppressing natural urges[3]. On the contrary, it is an essential function in all healthy people. It is worth examining this concept in more detail.

It used to be thought that, when you intend to make a movement, your brain just had to send a message via the nervous system to the muscles concerned, saying, in effect, 'Come on, wake up, get busy!' Nowadays, scientists know that an equally important function of the brain and nervous system is that of restraining muscles until the proper moment. This does not mean either 'relaxing' them or 'holding them back'. It simply means not suggesting action to them in the first place. In the passage quoted above, Sherrington was explaining that, whether we know it or not, a great deal of brain activity goes into *not* activating muscles.

This is significant, indeed of immense practical importance to us all. We should be well-advised to think of moving as a matter of *giving permission* to the muscles concerned, rather than of spurring them into action. Between these two approaches, there is all the difference between, let us say, letting a lively young dog off the lead, and whipping an unwilling donkey.

In fact, our muscles are only too ready and willing to get into action – the problem is one of selection. We should think of precision of movement as a matter of withholding permission from certain muscles, of asking them not to act. There are important nuances here: a young dog pulling at the lead is not obeying you as your muscles ought to obey you. You can control him to some extent by pulling at the lead yourself, but this is tiring and tedious. How much pleasanter to have a well-trained dog walking to heel without a lead, ready and willing to run and fetch! The quiet authority of the good dog trainer, the obedient and happy alertness of the well-trained dog, supply the model for the desirable relationship between mind and muscle.

As we know, even a good dog may sometimes be tempted to run or jump up at the wrong time – then, just *before* he starts to move, he needs a friendly reminder that you expect him to continue to behave himself. So do our muscles need such reminders. Of course, it is easier to check the dog when you first see the idea coming into his head, rather than when he has already started to do what you don't want him to do! And so it is with your own muscles. The process that neurologists call *inhibition* is supposed to be dealt with by the brain and nervous system and not by the muscles themselves.

Let us take a concrete example. Suppose you are learning the violin and you are (understandably) a bit afraid of dropping it when the left hand has awkward things to do. So perhaps you use muscles to raise your shoulder, so as to try to get a better grip. Your teacher, rightly, tells you that the shoulder should not be raised. Now what happens? You want to do as your teacher suggests – but habit is strong and somehow your shoulder keeps lifting. So you *hold* it down by muscle power. Now it looks more like what the teacher meant – but it isn't really. Things are still not working very well because now you are doubly interfering with your shoulder, by simultaneously trying to lift it and to hold it down! Until you stop doing both these things, your arm will not function as freely as it should, the violinistic problem will remain unsolved – and you will probably not be very comfortable either. The answer is: true inhibition, prevention of the original fault – so that there is nothing to 'correct'.

It is worth asking ourselves how good we are at letting our muscles know *when not to get in on the act*. This is an important question, for on this capacity depends our power to make choices, our freedom to explore our abilities and increase our skill.

Many of my readers will have seen on TV that great pianist, the late Arthur Rubinstein. Have you ever wondered how he could make everything look so easy, even when he was ninety years of age? We have already seen that waffling on about 'relaxation' merely avoids the question. The answer is that the best performers in any field are those whose co-ordination makes it possible for them to choose precisely when, where and how much to allow muscles to contract, and when to withhold that permission. Perhaps they can't explain how, but they are able to be truly selective. They not only know how to do what they want to do; more fundamentally, they also know how *not* to do anything that would get in the way of what they want to achieve.

We all have this faculty and constantly make use of it to a large extent. In fact, a great part of our brain is devoted to this 'choosing-not-to' type of control – so much so that we tend to take it for granted. It is easier to appreciate its vital importance if you consider what life is like for someone who has suffered damage to those parts of the brain that normally make these essential 'negative' choices. Such people have difficulty in accomplishing *any* action, because the instant they decide to move some part of them, *everything* starts to move. Imagine trying to thread a needle, do up a button, or even put your gloves on, if both your arms would insist on moving all over the place. Imagine being unable to move your mouth to form the one word 'Yes' without nearly jumping off your chair. Imagine being seized by spasms which painfully twist you into contortions against your will. Imagine being unable to put on the light because these contortions prevent your hand from getting near the switch. These things *really happen* to people in whom some part of the 'choosing-not-to' (i.e. inhibitory) mechanism has broken down and who therefore cannot be selective in their movements.

Between the misery and frustration of such sufferers on the one hand, and on the other the ease and mastery of a Rubinstein, we may picture a sort of sliding scale on which we place all the fairly ordinary people: you, me, little Jimmy who drops everything, Auntie whose knitting is so smooth, that pretty girl stumbling slightly as she walks, the fat man with the surprisingly light footsteps, the butcher confidently handling his dangerous tools – all imaginable degrees of skill or clumsiness that we class as 'normal'. We can see ourselves as moving up and down this scale according to how well we manage not to do the things that may interfere with our intentions.

Scientists tell us that we all have a lot of unused brain cells. If we can wake up some of those cells that are lazing about in the 'choosing-not-to' areas, we shall become more efficient movers, less frustrated, more confident, happier, healthier people. But how to wake up those cells? How to increase our power to think effectively in this respect?

Some pointers are given as this book proceeds. They will mean much more to you if you work through the intervening explanations first. As you do so, it will be good to place each explanation and each experiment within as realistic an image of yourself as you can build up. Muscularly speaking, the choices available to each of us are astronomical. However, not only are our nerves and muscles capable of acting very rapidly, they would rather like to do so according to patterns already familiar to them. In the absence of clear instructions from us, they will probably do this time what they have done before.

To by-pass this tendency is a real triumph of imagination. All our lives, people have been telling us *what to do*. Even when they say 'not like that', they usually add, in a stronger voice, 'Like **this**'. And we, hurrying to get it right, often fail to see that *not like that* is an indispensable precondition of *like this*. What's more, we adopt a similar way of giving instructions to ourselves, pushing ourselves to get something done, without giving much thought to what should be avoided – behaving to ourselves like an impatient boss. But we could instead adopt towards ourselves the role of parents who love to see the toddler's awakening capacities, who welcome each discovery with excitement, who react to each set-back with patience. Only think of the astonishing amount of learning that children achieve in the first few years of life! All this accomplishment would be impossible if they were hustled along, not allowed to make mistakes, not given time to experiment.

Learn from the way you treat your children. Whenever you want to improve the way you do something, give *yourself* plenty of time to experiment. If something is difficult, before you make greater efforts, even before you start thinking what to do, be ready to wonder if you are already doing something that increases the difficulty. Above all, give yourself time to say 'supposing I see to it that I *don't...*' whatever element you have decided temporarily to set aside.

We all have a tendency to want to arrive at conclusions, and this puts us in danger of trying to act on hypotheses that are mutually contradictory. Mentally and muscularly, no experiment can be made by someone who is not prepared to abandon some assumptions. By understanding the importance of getting things out of the way, of clearing the decks before getting to work, you have already begun the job.

---

1. Gray's *Anatomy*, p. 746 (Introduction to Neurology).
2. C. Sherrington, *The Brain and its Mechanism*, Rede Lecture, Cambridge University, 1933 (C.U.P.) quoted in *Selected Writings of Sir Charles Sherrington*, ed. D. Denny-Brown (O.U.P., 1979).
3. *Oxford English Dictionary:* 'By *inhibition* we mean the arrest of the functions of a structure or organ, by the action on it of another, while its power to execute those functions is still retained. L. Brunton *(Nature*, 1st March, 1883)'.
   This, the physiological meaning of the word, is also the 'most frequent meaning' according to the 1977 *Shorter O.E.D.*, which does not mention any 'psychological' or 'colloquial' sense. It is essential to bear this in mind when reading Alexander.

PART IV
ESSENTIAL INFORMATION
(specific)

CHAPTER 11

ABOUT BREATHING

... the air itself ... worth all the pearls and diamonds in ten thousand worlds ...
by reason of its precious and pure transparency, that all worlds would be nothing
without such a treasure...

Thomas Traherne *Centuries*

Continuing our work of clearing away possible misunderstandings, we now enter upon
an area where this tidying up process is most urgently needed: that is, the whole matter
of breathing. I can think of few aspects of life where we are so vulnerable to superstition.

The way we breathe is really a by-product of the way we manage the framework. Unfortunately, it quite often happens, when I am trying to explain something about the
framework, that people run ahead of me and start to talk about breathing. But now that
we have discussed the framework and some of the influences acting upon it, this seems a
good moment to look carefully at some of the most prevalent assumptions that beset any
discussion of breathing. I should like to ask for your 'willing suspension of disbelief' until my argument is complete. In talking about breathing, we face a special difficulty –
that language is linear, one word after another. Yet here, above all, we are dealing with
things that are far from linear: things interdependent, contained in each other, often virtually simultaneous.

Having read the discussion in Chapter 10, perhaps you will not be surprised to find
that much of the practical advice I have to give (and it *is* practical) will be of an apparently
negative nature – suggesting what *not* to do. As Alexander emphasized, for the right thing
to do itself, we need to stop doing the wrong thing. But sadly, so much of what we have
been taught, or have assumed without being taught it, is under the influence of the kind of
thinking that says: 'If something is wrong – quick! do the opposite and that must be right.'
Those might well be the words of a spell cast on us in infancy by some wicked fairy who
wished to put a blight on our whole life. For if we see 'right' as the opposite of 'wrong', we
are condemned for ever to fly from one extreme to the other – and the moment when we
pass through the 'happy medium' is so brief that we scarcely notice its existence. Nowhere
is this more true than in the much-discussed matter of breathing.

You might think that when people start telling you how you ought to do something
which in any case nature obliges you to do continuously from birth to death, you could

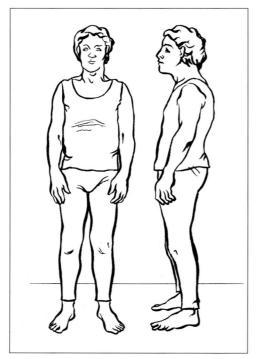

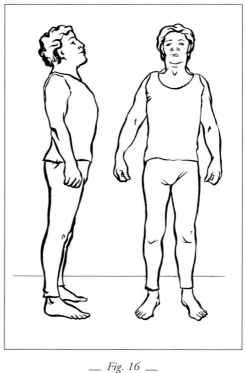

— *Fig. 15* —

All squashed up, with chest collapsed

— *Fig. 16* —

Sometimes thought of as 'taking a deep breath', but it is nothing of the sort.

justifiably tell them where to go with their advice! Yet lots of people allow other people to tell them that they are not breathing properly. They will even accept ideas about how they ought to breathe, and try to put such ideas into practice, without ever questioning whether their mentors know any more about it than they do themselves, or can prove themselves any better at it. I find this amazing.

Most of the confusion about breathing stems from the fact that, although nearly all the time it is supposed to be automatic and self-regulating, it is also necessary that we should *just occasionally* be able to interfere with the natural process – for instance when passing through thick smoke. We humans are apt to be so proud of the conscious part of our brain that we jump to the conclusion that anything we can bring under its control will necessarily be improved. This is a fallacy. *The only way we can consciously improve on the functioning of our automatic or quasi-automatic processes is by removing interference and giving them room and opportunity to function.*

Confusion is further confounded by the fact that breathing is so essential to survival that nature has provided us with several fail-safe systems. Just as we can breathe through the mouth when the nose is blocked, so there are a number of different possible movements that will result in air entering and leaving the lungs. Some ways are more energy-efficient than others – but obviously even the worst way is better than not breathing at all!

So much depends on circumstances. Normal breathing is a combination of movements of the ribs and diaphragm. (**Chapter 4**) The way the responsibility is shared varies according to total body attitude. Some examples: lying on the back somewhat restricts rib movement and so the diaphragm has to do a greater proportion of the work; leaning a long way forward in a sitting position (as you might when doing up your shoes) increases pressure within the abdomen, thus limiting diaphragm movement – so the ribs are therefore obliged to take up more of the work. If, in an accident, you were squashed in a space where the movement of both ribs and diaphragm were seriously restricted, you would be only too glad to breathe by using muscles in your neck to raise and lower your chest – an exhausting procedure which in normal circumstances would be regarded as a symptom of illness[1]. These are just some of the more obvious examples of the possible variations within that subtle and complex process we know as breathing.

If ever there was a case for saying 'nature knows best' it is in this matter of breathing. In nature, breathing is regulated by the total activity of the moment (i.e. according to the working muscles' demand for oxygen from the blood) and by the physical attitude of the framework, which determines by what breathing movements that demand can be satisfied.

Now obviously, if you are all squashed up with your chest collapsed (fig. 15), there will not be much room for breath in your lungs, so when you need more air you will be obliged to lift up the chest – or (more probably, if you have got into this mess in the first place) you will *tilt* your chest, raising it in front by hollowing your back. In that case, when you breathe out you will collapse and round your back again. This is what many people call 'taking a deep breath' (fig. 16). It is nothing of the sort. The hollowing of the back restricts the movement of the lower ribs and interferes with the functioning of the diaphragm, rendering a 'deep breath' impossible.

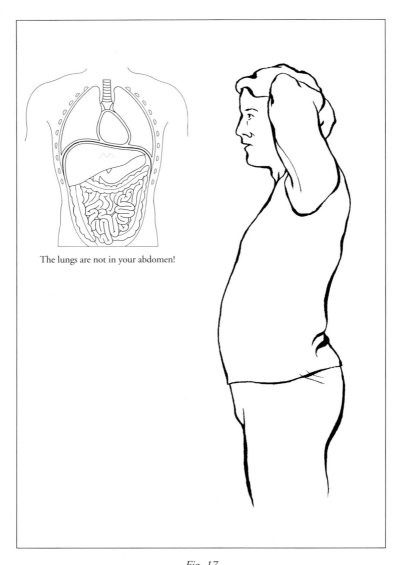

The lungs are not in your abdomen!

— Fig. 17 —
'Abdominal' breathing restricts rib movement.

In reaction against this sort of thing (remember what I said about people flying to extremes?) some people advocate what they call 'abdominal breathing'. (The expression is rather absurd – I need hardly point out that the only place for breath to go is into your lungs – and they are certainly not in your abdomen!) What is called 'abdominal' breathing involves a downwards compression of the abdominal organs, resulting in a visible swelling of the abdominal region. It is physiologically impossible without restricting rib freedom (fig. 17).

The abdominal muscles do have a part to play in breathing. However, the marked bulging on the in-breath, of which some people are so proud, merely indicates a weak abdominal wall – the weakness usually having been induced by deliberate practice of this style of breathing. The advocates of 'abdominal breathing' are sometimes quite hard to shake because they believe that there is something spiritual about their breathing pattern. You can see a similar style of breathing in some badly-taught singers and players of wind instruments. *They* like to call it 'diaphragmatic breathing' – but are often vague about what they mean by the expression. (There are even some very good singers who use a similar approach and – thanks to a combination of talent and a strong physique – get away with it, for a considerable time in some cases.)

On one of my courses, I met a young woman who told me she had been on a course about breathing and therefore knew all about it. Though unable to say *what* the diaphragm is, nor *where* it is, still less how it works, she considered it part of her job to teach her little recorder pupils to 'breathe with their diaphragms' – and had apparently no qualms about her meddling. Such abuse of a teacher's influence, and of a child's trust, is a real danger to health; alas, it is not uncommon.

F.M. Alexander, discussing ill-advised respiratory education, notes:

> ... when the diaphragm is unduly depressed in inspiration ... there is a sinking above and below the clavicles, a hollowing in the lumbar region of the back, undue protrusion of the abdomen, displacement of the abdominal viscera, reduction in height, undue depression of the larynx...[2]

Dr Pierre Bonnier also issues the direst warnings against this aberration, citing:

> the danger (to women even more than to men) of compressing, distorting and even displacing a whole list of organs: kidneys, intestines, bladder, womb and ovaries.[3]

A friend of mine has yet another name for this type of breathing: she calls it 'abdominable' (sic) breathing – probably the best name of all for it!

Of course, nothing that I have said here alters the fact that in certain positions you will notice slight abdominal movement during breathing. There is nothing fancy about this. One of the things that occur during a normal in-breath is that the diaphragm and ribs collaborate to create space in the thorax, allowing incoming air to expand the lungs. During this phase of breathing, the diaphragm is pressing down on the contents of the abdomen, lest they should try to occupy the increased thoracic space designed for the incoming air. (fig. 18) The abdominal contents in turn, therefore, naturally press on the muscular wall of the abdomen, tending to stretch it and cause *slight* bulging.

At this point, in a person whose 'carriage' is good, that is, whose framework maintains its expanded state (**Chapters 7/8/17/24**) the abdominal muscles will automatically

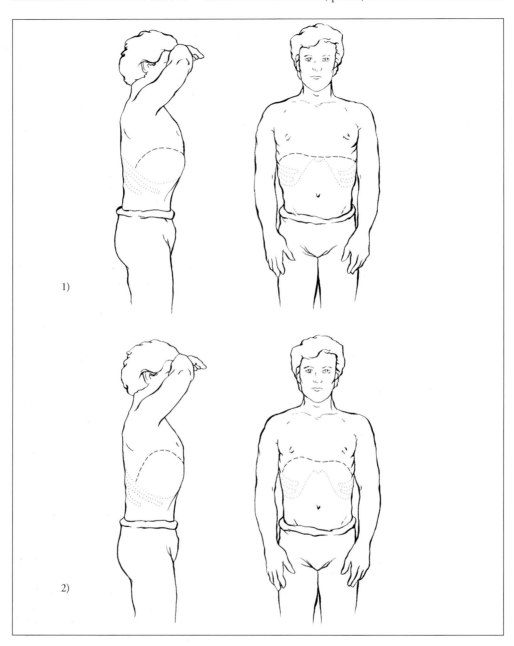

1)

2)

— *Fig. 18* —

Broken line shows level of diaphragm.
1) after breathing in; 2) after breathing out.

resist the stretch that is being placed upon them. Stretch reflexes (**Chapter 7**) are involved here, stimulated also by the sideways lift of the ribs natural to the in-breath. This reflex reaction limits the displacement of the viscera. What one notices, therefore, in a well co-ordinated person, is a change in the activity and tonus of the abdominal muscles, rather than any marked abdominal bulging.

The reflex reaction I have just described has an important part to play in singing. It is the essential foundation of what good singers mean when they talk about 'supporting the breath'. But then, the best singers always work with an expanded framework. This cannot always be said of their pupils, which is why explanations about 'support' are often woefully misunderstood. The root of the misunderstanding lies in the reflex nature of the process: within an expanding framework, when a big demand is placed on the organism, these reflex workings can be strongly felt and the teacher will naturally attempt to describe such feelings. Of course, it is valid to do so. However, no amount of trying – or of trying to feel – will bring about the correct reflex response in the pupil if the framework is partially collapsed.

When the condition of the framework does not allow of proper 'abdominal support' for the breath, I have even heard of singing teachers adopting a solution so misconceived that it is quite fascinating: the pupil, who by the wrong sort of *trying* to work his abdominal muscles has abused them to the point where they are incapable of efficient work (**Chapter 7**) is now recommended to wear a stout corset! By such means does man try to 'improve' on the wonderful gifts of nature. (As I have said, the fact that exceptional individuals succeed while ignoring nature's rules should not encourage anyone to underestimate the price that nature can exact for such meddling.)

There is another trap into which people can easily fall – more understandably but none the less dangerously. It consists of holding the ribs fixed in their widened position, by which I mean the place they would naturally occupy at the end of a normal in-breath. People who have had lessons in the Alexander Technique sometimes fall into this trap, if they have not really grasped what is meant by 'widening the back'. If not corrected, this tendency leads to a stiffened rib-cage, one less able to adapt itself with ease to the body's oxygen requirements. Again, some singers and actors commit this interference with nature quite deliberately, perhaps believing that the breath will not last unless they do something about it. (Of course, without a suitable framework, this is true: *something* will have to be done!)

It is also important to know that, despite 'folk-lore' to the contrary, it is impossible to empty your lungs completely. The quantity of air that stays in them all the time is considerably greater than the amount of tidal air that comes and goes when you are breathing quietly.[4] So if your breathing organ has not become inefficient through repeated misuse, you can usually find a little more breath if you really need it. Suppose you were crossing a busy street and saw your friend about to step in front of a bus – I doubt if you would waste time going through the performance of 'taking a deep breath' before shouting 'look out!'

In fact, the whole idea of *taking* a breath (deep or otherwise) is perhaps the greatest of all the many misunderstandings about breathing. It certainly is the point of departure for the creation of innumerable unnecessary problems. Whenever you *notice* someone breathing in, whether what catches your attention is the little gasp affected by TV newsreaders before they say 'Good evening' (and indeed before practically every sentence they utter) or the sniffing sound people make when they are conscientiously breathing in the lovely fresh air through their noses, you may be sure that what they are really doing is impeding the free flow of air to the lungs! The sniff or gasp is the audible proof that the air passage is being narrowed. It is so obvious, if you think about it, that it is almost laughable.

There is nothing you can *do* to breathe in that does not make breathing in more difficult. If you have breathed out, you will certainly breathe in. You have no choice in the matter as long as you live. But by messing about with this process a lot of people manage to make life extremely uncomfortable for themselves. If I could pass one law, it would be this: nobody would be allowed to say 'take a deep breath'. (I might be persuaded to make an exception for doctors when using a stethoscope – but I should love to know how vets manage!)

If the framework is right and if you don't interfere, your breathing will always adapt itself to the needs of the activity you are performing. This may sound a daring statement but the truth of it has been proved with singers and players of wind instruments. Encouraging results are usually obtained quite quickly once the principle has been grasped and accepted. *If the framework is not in good condition, trying to be clever about breathing will only make both framework and breathing worse than they are already.*

Furthermore, it is axiomatic that if a system is in need of correction and improvement, any demand placed on it will tend to exacerbate the fault. The greater the demand, the greater the risk. (You know this is true of your car.) So here is one very important piece of advice: **don't do breathing exercises!** They will only exaggerate any existing faults in your breathing pattern. In my teaching experience, this is true even of such apparently non-invasive techniques as awareness exercises (where people are encouraged 'only to observe' the breathing). **(See Chapter 12.)**

If you are perfect, you don't need breathing exercises; if you are not perfect, be warned against them. They can even create problems. I might quote the case of my own father, whose youthful enthusiasm for breathing exercises did not prevent him from becoming, in later life, one of the worst asthmatics ever seen. Indeed, it seems to me that his past attempts to 'improve' his breathing contributed to his illness. I certainly observed that his breathing was freer whenever his frantic efforts to breathe exhausted him to the point where he lost consciousness. The tragic fact was that he simply could not allow nature to get on with a job that belongs to her own domain – and this I attribute partly to the fact that he had conscientiously practised interfering with the natural process. He died at sixty-one of heart failure brought on by his appalling struggles to do the most natural thing in the world, namely to allow the air that is our permanent surrounding element to leave and re-enter his body.

His was an extreme and clear-cut case of something one often sees in modified form. Since I am being autobiographical for the moment, I should tell you that I was considerably affected by seeing what I have described. As a young adult I developed a similar pattern of struggle when confronted with life's difficulties. Breathing thus became problematical for me also, until at last I learnt some common sense about it. Please, don't try to teach your children to 'breathe properly' – the answer lies elsewhere.

'But', you may say, 'I am conscious that, for whatever reason, my breathing is not as it should be. Surely there is something I can do about it?' Well, yes, there is, but before I can explain it, it is absolutely necessary for us to get rid of misunderstandings. So let us take a look at what is really supposed to happen in natural breathing.

As you know, breathing enables the body to receive oxygen, by passing it from the lungs to the blood. A similar exchange takes place when carbon dioxide from the blood passes into the lungs and is exhaled. The body's need for oxygen is greater during energetic exercise than at other times; during exercise there is also more carbon dioxide to be got rid of. That is why when we exercise we tend to breathe more deeply; and why, if the exercise is unaccustomed, we pant. This reaction is automatic, of course. It would be well-nigh impossible to overrule it. This is because the brain is kept constantly informed of the balance of oxygen to carbon dioxide in the blood. The brain acts on information received, constantly adapting the instructions it gives the breathing mechanism as to the speed of breathing and the volume of air to be displaced. All this is so well known that it is not easy to understand how anyone ever got the idea that 'deep breathing' was a good thing in itself, that divorcing it from the activity that should induce it could achieve any beneficial results. The reverse is the case. *Deep breathing exercises are always risky and usually harmful.*

Early in the twentieth century, appalling things were done in the name of deep breathing (fig. 19). Fortunately, the worst of the craze has passed by now. However, it has left quite a number of people with a guilty feeling that they really ought to breathe more deeply. They are often relieved to learn that the deep-breathing superstition was just another example of the human tendency to mistrust the body's ability to know its own business. One wonders why anyone ever supposed it to be a good thing to breathe deeply when not engaged in activity demanding a large supply of oxygen. In fact, to do so upsets the chemical balance of the bloodstream. (As a child you may have found out that you could make yourself dizzy by over-breathing.) Abusing nature in this way would be very dangerous, were it not for the fact that there is a fail-safe mechanism: a person who persisted too long would faint until the balance had been restored. Even so, the procedure is not to be recommended!

Perhaps the deep-breathing myth arose from a real concern for the health of people crowded in offices and factories, stooping or slumping, tired and fed up. Of course it is good to get out, move, breathe fresh air – we need all this for many reasons. A good brisk walk induces more lively breathing – but to activate the breathing without the walk is more dubious. It was a grave mistake to take *just one aspect* of well-being and single it out for interference.

Each of us is provided with an 'automatic pilot' for round-the-clock adaptation of complex breathing movements to oxygen demand. Attempts to improve on this precision equipment are worse than pointless. If the equipment seems faulty the explanation is often that someone has been fooling about with it.

The first and most necessary step is to stop meddling!

(For the professional use of the voice, there are teachers who know exactly how to prepare a pupil's breathing organ for demands about to be placed on it. They usually

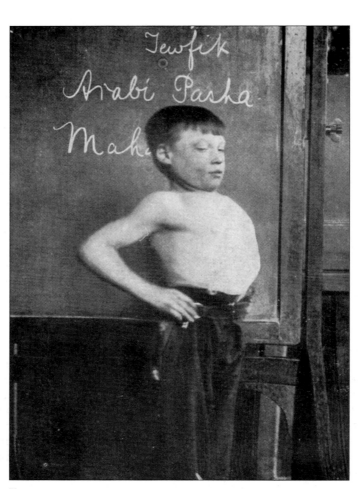

THIS PHOTOGRAPH, PUBLISHED A FEW YEARS AGO IN AN ENGLISH DAILY PAPER, REPRESENTS A MEMBER OF A CLASS IN A LONDON COUNTY COUNCIL SCHOOL PERFORMING DEEP BREATHING EXERCISES. ON THE BACK OF THIS PAGE THIS LAD MAY BE SEEN AT WORK IN THE CLASS. THESE UNFORTUNATE BOYS AS HERE SHOWN ARE SIMPLY BEING DEVELOPED INTO DEFORMITIES. LUCKILY OF LATE A CHANGE FOR THE BETTER HAS BEEN TAKEN PLACE IN SCHOOL CALISTHENICS.

— *Fig. 19* —

Appalling things were done in the name of deep breathing ... and were strongly criticized by F.M. Alexander in his first book.

manage to do this in a surprisingly short time and without fuss: not by exercises as normally understood but by a carefully controlled awakening of the whole organ to its own subtleties and strengths. Unless you are being supervised by one of these rare experts, it will be far better for you to have nothing to do with any breathing exercises whatsoever. I cannot sufficiently stress that even the most apparently harmless have their dangers.)

Having got all that out of the way, we can return to the question you may still be asking: 'What can I do to improve my breathing?' Firstly, if you feel that your breathing is in need of improvement, do some kind of regular physical activity that appeals to you for its own sake. If you are doing something *for fun*, you are less likely to have attention to spare for any nonsense about regulating your breathing; and nature will normally see to it that you get the additional oxygen you need, provided you do not push yourself into doing more than you are capable of and feel like doing. Athletes are well aware of the 'training effect' – the organism's gradual adaption to gradually increasing demands – so be patient. (**More about exercise in Chapter 31.**)

If the training effect does not seem to be working for you, if you always get quickly out of breath during exercise, or if your 'quiet breathing' (when you are doing nothing in particular) still seems rather agitated, you might try the following procedure. *I must emphasize that this is not an exercise but an experiment in non-interference.* (Alexander teachers will notice that I have in this instance adapted Alexander's preferred 'experiment'. I have done so because, in my experience, people tend to notice resemblances to familiar exercises, whereas subtle but important differences tend to be overlooked.)

❏ *Experiment*

Without interrupting whatever breathing rhythm you happen to have on the go at the time, and *without taking a special breath* (not even that little extra you often take before starting to speak – be strict with yourself about this or the experiment will not be valid) next time you just happen to be breathing out, make a little noise: if you can easily roll your 'r's (at the front of the mouth, Scottish style, not like a French 'r') then 'rrrrrrr' is very good for this experiment; otherwise use that vibration of the lips that children make when imitating a motor-bike. Both can be done with voice or in a sort of whisper. It really helps a lot if you can pretend to yourself that you are making the sound to attract the attention of a kitten or to amuse a small child. *Don't squeeze the air out* – there are no prizes for length, and if you make hard work of it you can't expect the reflex to work properly. Make your chosen noise until such time as you would rather like to breathe in again. At that moment, *close your mouth and deliberately turn your mind to something else* – your plans for tomorrow, a picture on the wall, a headline in the paper, anything will do as long as it is not particularly loaded emotionally. Best of all, think about your head being free to balance itself. (**Chapter 14**) Sooner or later, air will come into your lungs.

It is not up to you to decide whether the air comes at once or after a pause. It doesn't matter whether it comes quickly or slowly, a lot or a little. The whole point is to leave such decisions to reflexes in your body, which know much more about these things than you could ever know. Above all, don't be tempted to 'top up' – make do with the air your body decides to admit on this particular occasion.

Air will come in easily through your nose, unless you have such a bad cold that both nostrils are completely blocked. One might say, indeed, that two nostrils are a luxury, for the air passage inside your nose is much wider than it looks – as long as you don't narrow it by a sniffing action. A useful antidote to sniffing is that flaring of the nostrils that occurs high up, around the bridge of the nose – you can identify it when you want to laugh at the wrong moment: a tiny reaction that facilitates breathing, and is encouraged when you see the funny side of things. (If your glasses restrict it, get them adjusted.) Air intake via the nose is preferable whenever possible: by taking that route, the air gets filtered and warmed, and so is less likely to cause irritation.

Do not carry out this procedure more than three or four times in a row. Make the same experiment in different positions and during various activities: slumped on a sofa, standing upright, cleaning the bath, looking straight ahead, looking up at the ceiling, walking, all the variations you can think of. But only a little at a time. Remember, you are not looking for any particular rhythm. Play with your noises, have fun with them as children do. It will help to distract you from your in-breath.

When you have made this experiment a few times, you may allow yourself to be *mildly* interested in the length of your noises. (But still ignore your breathing in!) You will probably notice that some of your noises last longer than others. If so, good. If not, you are interfering somehow and had better stop even this little experiment. It doesn't necessarily mean that you interfere when you *don't* think about it.

Whether or not the above experiment has proved useful for you, you might try sometimes, when you are working hard or thinking about something with great concentration, just asking yourself if you are holding your breath in. People often do so without noticing. If you find that you are, don't do anything special about it; just quietly give yourself permission to breathe out. *The next in-breath will follow of its own accord, sooner or later* – and who is in a hurry?

Or perhaps, on the contrary, you tend to hold your breath *out* when you are absorbed? There is still nothing special to be done, as we usually understand doing. In any kind of breathing difficulty, the best advice is first to say to yourself that no anxiety – about breathing or anything else – shall interfere with the freedom of the head to balance itself; then gently allow your body to take up as much room in the world as its comfort requires. The breathing will probably adjust itself, and air will come to occupy the space created by your expanding framework. There is enough air for everybody and nothing to be gained by snatching at it greedily. You would think it rude to snatch at food – there is even less reason to be in a rush to get at the air!

One reason why breathing is difficult to write about is that authorities differ as to what exactly does take place! The 1973 edition of Gray's *Anatomy*, that essential reference work, tells us of a variety of opinions concerning the action of the intercostal muscles (muscles which connect adjacent ribs) and adds: 'These controversies have not yet been resolved'. Of another set of muscles (*levatores costarum*) it says that 'they elevate the ribs but their importance in respiration is disputed'.[5] (Later editions raise other questions.) I am told that Husler, who studied anatomical texts in several languages when preparing his book on the physiology of singing, found that the muscle *transversus thoracis*, on which great importance was placed by Italian authorities, received decreasing attention the further north one went, virtually disappearing in the Scandinavian texts he consulted!

One understands the difficulty encountered by physiologists in attempting a general description of breathing. To quote Gray's again:

> The range and character of the movements (of the chest wall) exhibit very striking variations, which may be dependent on the conformation of the thoracic skeleton, *on habit or on other factors*, and this extreme variability must be borne in mind when the movements are being analysed in any particular subject. (My italics)[6]

However, all is not lost. We can ask ourselves how the physiologists went about reaching their (tentative) conclusions. Presumably they examined a number of people who happened to be available. But, as Maslow says:

> If we want to answer the question how tall can the human species grow, then obviously it is well to pick out the ones who are already tallest and study them. If we want to know how fast a human being can run, then it is no use to average out the speed of 'a good sample' of the population; it is far better to collect Olympic gold-medal winners and see how well they can do.[7]

Similarly, if we want to know about breathing, it is no bad idea to take note of people who are demonstrably good at it. Failure to discriminate in this way may account for discrepancies in the (no doubt reliable) observations reported by various authorities.

Let us therefore take for consideration three writers whose claim to our attention rests on their own performance or that of their pupils, or both.

1) Just before the turn of the century, a young actor was having problems with loss of voice associated with audible breathing. After a long period of self-observation and self re-education (a fascinating story well worth studying in detail) he became famous, particularly for his breath control in demanding Shakespearian roles – so much so that other actors demanded lessons and leading doctors sent him their patients for respiratory re-education. He was Frederick Matthias Alexander (1869-1955), founder of the now well-known Alexander Technique and teacher of the greatest names in the theatre of his day. (**See Chapter 34.**)

What did such a man have to say on the subject of breathing? Of all things, he maintained that *breathing as such does not exist*: it is a by-product of the total co-ordination, dependent on the shape and activity of the body at any given moment. He wrote that

> ... so-called 'bad breathing' is only a symptom and not a primary cause ... we are mistaking a general malcondition for a specific defect ... the standard of breathing depends on the standard of general co-ordinated use of the psycho-physical mechanisms.[8]

2) Compare this with what Frederick Husler, well-known singing teacher and author of *Singen: Die physische Natur des Stimmorganes* (1965) had to say about what he called the 'respiratory scaffolding':

> If one considers the delicately adjusted dynamic in which the act of expiration in singing has to take place, the obvious conclusion seems to be that some kind of framework must exist within which the breathing mechanism can carry out its work with perfect freedom of action. Such a scaffolding is recognizable in the combined action of a number of trunk muscles, from which the expiratory mechanism is, as it were, suspended.[9]

He adds that this scaffolding

> cannot be acquired by 'fixing', 'adjusting' or 'holding' – it is fashioned only by correct movement.[10]

Alexander and Husler were not in contact but were agreed that, if the framework were properly maintained during exhalation, the in-breath would follow of its own accord and needed no attention.

Why the discrepancy between this and the emphasis so often placed on the act of breathing *in*? Many people seem to take the view, expressed by Basmajian, that 'although inspiration is a muscular effort, expiration is an elastic recoil'.[11] Physiotherapists among my pupils often tell me that such is the basis on which they have been taught to 're-educate' people's breathing. When asked what they mean by this very incomplete description, they demonstrate a lifting and tilting of the rib-cage during the in-breath, followed by a sort of collapse of the whole trunk on breathing out – i.e. a folding at the waist, combined with a lowering of the breast-bone. This may not be what Basmajian meant, but such is the way in which an already far too prevalent fault receives as it were official status! Alexander remarked scornfully of this procedure, 'This isn't breathing; it's lifting your chest and collapsing'.

Husler's description of breathing is based on the 'respiratory scaffolding' working 'with maximum efficiency in the few great singers who emerge from time to time' and whom he advises us to take as 'models to be attentively observed'.[12] I submit that what is observed in great singers, who give daily proof of the efficiency of what they are doing, is more worthy of our attention than any mere account of what is seen to occur in people who are only 'normal' in the sense of not being actually ill at the moment. Note that I say, 'what is *observed*'. We must be cautious in accepting great singers' *descriptions* of what they do. What is obvious to them may not be so to us and hence their words may cause confusion.

3) Another source which merits interest is Dr Pierre Bonnier's book, which I have already quoted. (We can refer to Bonnier, as to Husler, without involvement in singers' polemics. What matters here is that the passages quoted are strikingly in agreement with Alexander's teaching and with my own observations.) Bonnier's work came to my attention a few years ago when I heard that a singer named Alice Thieffry had won acclaim for a solo performance in Brussels Cathedral *on the eve of her ninety-nineth birthday!* I finally obtained an introduction to this remarkable lady who had continued singing some forty years beyond the usual retirement age – only to find that she had just died, aged a hundred. A friend kindly assuaged my frustration by obtaining for me a copy of Bonnier's book (long out of print), to which Miss Thieffry had declared she owed her radiant and accomplished old age. Her health had been very bad when she was young, but she loved singing, and this book was the starting point of her transformation.

Bonnier's account of the intricate interplay of forces operating on the organ of breathing – long, technical, closely argued, sometimes controversial – goes beyond our purposes here, but the following is worth quoting:

> ... thoracic expansion adapts itself to all the body's attitudes and varies at each instant. The respiratory

style thus varies at every moment and it would be preposterous to demand uniform movement from an organ which changes shape, which must accommodate itself to variable hindrances and take advantage of equally variable scope. One attitude permits a mode of breathing that another attitude will prohibit and it is thoroughly absurd to wish to fix a rule which will be broken at every moment by the necessity of breathing in a convenient and serviceable way in the most diverse positions and movements.[13] (My translation)

I have gone into all this at some length because, as de Bono says, 'it is not the ideas we do not have that block our thinking but the ideas that we do have'.

How does breathing work when you habitually use your framework in its expanding mode? Adequate description is not easy, but, with balanced muscle use of the trunk, what happens is roughly as follows. The spinal column being neither collapsed nor exaggeratedly arched, the ribs can move about it to play their part in expelling air or letting it into the lungs. The shoulder girdle (consisting of shoulder-blades and collar-bones) maintains its width back and front, so the breastbone remains in place, no longer rising on the in-breath and falling on the out-breath. (Indeed, in strong exhalation executed under ideal conditions, the breastbone tends to rise slightly in reaction to the rib movement.) Instead of sinking in an attempt to squash air from the chest cavity, and then being laboriously hauled up again to make room for the next lot of air, the breastbone, like the spine, acts as a stable basis for free rib movement. Each rib, according to its particular design, has room (within the limits dictated by the total body movement of the moment) to follow the route prescribed by nature, thanks to the gliding movements of the ribs where they articulate with the vertebrae.

Thus, during the in-breath, when each rib has the opportunity to follow its natural path, the total result is, essentially, *a lateral expansion of the ribcage.* This not only helps to make room for the incoming air: it also creates extra space within the ribcage for viscera displaced by diaphragm activity[14]. (Bear in mind that the upper abdomen is contained within the ribcage – fig. 14.) *Downward* displacement of the viscera will encounter some resistance from stretch reflexes in the abdominal muscles. This all works naturally and freely when the expanding framework sees to it that there is enough room for everything, and when the forced bulging of the lower abdomen is no longer seen as an option.

Slight changes in the abdominal wall are a normal result of displacement – particularly when you are lying on your back – but in nature we are protected from exaggerated distension. For most normal purposes, the prevention of floppy collapse of the abdominal wall does not call for voluntary tension of the abdominal muscles, which would be as unnecessary and undesirable as voluntary relaxation or collapse. Nature is much cleverer than all that! *Only take care of the expanding framework and your reflexes will take care of the rest.*

In breathing out, as the abdominal muscles come into play more positively, but still reflexly, the resulting pressure from the contents of the abdomen assists in the upward movement of the 'dome' of the diaphragm. The diaphragm, its 'dome' rising to expel air, is held down at the edges by the action of the ribs. Being thus increasingly stretched as you breathe out, it becomes increasingly ready to contract (**stretch reflex, Chapter 7**) and thus to co-operate with the sideways lift of the ribs in making room for the next influx of air. Here we see how *the action of each set of muscles is contained and eventually reversed by the reaction it provokes in opposing muscles.* Throughout the respiratory cycle, the same sort of thing occurs elsewhere in ways too complex to detail here. You can see why I am so insistent on the importance of getting out of the way and letting things happen.

Thus we see that, under these ideal conditions, the famous 'elastic recoil' operates in breathing in. We see why this phase of the respiratory cycle can rightly be described as 'a process that needs no attention or conscious effort'. At last, we see that respiration, far from being a series of piston-like efforts ('in-out, in-out') becomes a process we could better illustrate by a wheel or a figure eight, *the exhalation preparing and causing the inhalation and vice versa.* No wonder even a baby can do it!

Of course there is muscular work involved, both in breathing out and in breathing in – but that is no concern of ours. Despite the fact that the muscles concerned are of the 'voluntary' type, which (as mentioned above) allows us in special circumstances to overrule automatic processes for a while, under normal conditions all is taken care of reflexly as long as we take care of the framework, the scaffolding. (**Chapters 14 and 17 contain important information about this.**)

So if what you want is the well-being that comes from problem-free and properly adapted breathing, I suggest that if you postpone any further respiratory experimentation until you have learned to maintain and improve the framework, you will probably then find that nothing much remains to be done about breathing as such – that it is indeed a by-product. And if you are a singer, actor, wind-player or athlete – or have other reasons for feeling that you have special requirements – do remember that any specialized technique that is not constructed on a basis of sound understanding of natural processes is a house built upon sand.

Here are three short quotations that sum up what I have been saying:

> For the singer (as for the non-singer) every part of the widespread organ has its own part to perform and, even more important, all parts have to work in an elastic, resilient interplay together as an organic unit. To over-emphasize one part means to disrupt the whole. Above all *primarily* there is no art in breathing.
> Husler[15]

> There is in the brain a spot which ... works the breathing movement of the chest. That spot is so responsive to the state of aeration of the blood that the slightest deficiency ... at once proportionately increases that action of the chest, and ventilates the lung more freely. There is thus a governor-system regulating the taking of breath ... operated chemically and on the self-regulating plan. As though that were not enough, there is a further regulation, self-operated mechanically.
> Sherrington[16]

> ... it is incorrect and harmful to speak of 'teaching a person to breathe'.
> F.M. Alexander[17]

---

1. The sternocleidomastoid muscles can act as auxiliary muscles of respiration, and can often be seen to operate as such in asthmatics.
2. F.M. Alexander, *The Theory and Practice of a New Method of Respiratory Re-education* (1907) reprinted in

F.M. Alexander, *Articles and Lectures*, London, Mouritz, 1995.

3. P. Bonnier, *La Voix – sa culture physiologique*, Alcan, 1910.
4. W.G. Sears, *Anatomy and Physiology for Nurses and Students of Human Biology*, London, Edward Arnold, 4th edition, 1965, p. 252.
5. Gray's *Anatomy*, p. 515.
6. *ibid.* p. 519.
7. A. Maslow, *The Farther Reaches of Human Nature*, Harmondsworth, Penguin (Pelican) 1973, p. 7.
8. F.M. Alexander, *Constructive Conscious Control of the Individual* (1923) London, STAT Books, 1997, p. 135.
9. F. Husler and Y. Rodd-Marling, *Singing: the physical nature of the vocal organ*, London, Hutchinson, revised edition. 1976, p. 34.
10. *ibid.* p. 35.
11. J.V. Basmajian, *Primary Anatomy*, Baltimore, Williams and Wilkins, 7th edition, 1976, p. 48.
12. F. Husler and Y. Rodd-Marling, *op. cit.*, p. 35.
13. P. Bonnier, *op. cit.*, p. 48.
14. Gray's *Anatomy* p. 421.
15. F. Husler and Y. Rodd-Marling, *op. cit.*, p. 48.
16. C. Sherrington, *Man on his Nature*, Cambridge University Press, 1940, p. 148.
17. F.M. Alexander, *op. cit.*, p. 138.

CHAPTER 12

BREATH AND SPIRIT

> how should tasting touching hearing seeing
> breathing any – lifted from the no
> of all nothing – human merely being
> doubt unimaginable You?
> E.E. Cummings

From the earliest times, it seems, people have pondered the mystery of the breath: invisible, intangible, without which we cease to be, it seems to imply innumerable questions about our very existence. It also raises questions about our relationship to all else that exists, so perhaps it is not surprising to find, in the literature of many religious and philosophical traditions, that words such as *breath, life, spirit, wind*, tend to overlap in meaning. (A footnote in the *New English Bible* says '*Wind* and *spirit* are translations of the same Greek word, which has both meanings.') We also find evidence of individuals who, reflecting on these questions, have reached profound insights, which they have sometimes tried to share.

Therein, it seems to me, lies a certain difficulty. Insights of this kind, however far-reaching, are subtle, and they come as experience, within the context of the totality of an individual life. Hence they are hard to explain verbally, for the very words seem to change their meaning, on their way to the listening ears. When the words are seized on by people who have not shared the experience, *insights* rapidly turn into *methods*. In the process, they inevitably lose much of their essence; at worst they become grossly distorted. Hence the warnings one finds, in every tradition, against methods and systems; hence the insistence on the imperative need for personal guidance.

Hence, too, my own distrust of breathing exercises. I have made clear my own point of view in the previous chapter and shall not reiterate it here. But since it often comes as rather a surprise, it seemed desirable to draw attention to the somewhat similar opinions expressed, with some insistence, by people living at the heart of very different traditions. Sometimes, in reviewing these opinions, it seems possible to trace the process of transformation of an *experience* into an *idea* and thence into a *system*.

Many Orthodox Christians know and love the Jesus Prayer, an invocation of the holy name in a prayer so brief that it can be repeated in the midst of the routine concerns of every day. 'Numerous writers have mentioned the physical aspects of the prayer, the breathing exercises, the attention which is paid to the beating of the heart and a number of other minor features ... Ancient and modern Fathers have dealt with the subject, always coming to the same conclusion: never to attempt the physical exercises without strict guidance by a spiritual father.'[1]

St Hesychius, writing in the sixth or seventh century, suggested that linking the prayer to one's breathing could bring effortless joy and peace, leading to a life of virtually continuous prayer. Many were touched by the beauty and simplicity of this idea – but in time it seems to have been elaborated and systematized. A fourteenth-century text gives detailed instructions about postures and about *regulating the breath to conform to the prayer*. Assuming the accuracy of translations, this seems like a distortion of the original. Perhaps it explains why the practice was discouraged as mechanical, and why we find a nineteenth-century Orthodox bishop advising against it, on the grounds that 'many people have harmed their lungs and achieved nothing'.[2]

The Sufi master Hazrat Inayat Khan, in emphasizing the importance of the breath in bringing 'order and harmony' to body, mind and soul, has this warning to give: 'There are many who without proper guidance and knowledge practise breath. Year after year they go on and very little result is achieved ... and very often the little veins of the brain and chest are ruptured by wrong breathing. There are many who have experienced this by not knowing how to breathe. One has to be extremely careful; one must do breathing practices rightly or not do them at all.'[3]

Gurdjieff was equally outspoken about breathing exercises. 'The risk is great (he is reported as saying) for the machine is very complicated ... If anyone here is experimenting with breathing, it is better to stop while there is still time.'[4] He explained that 'the difficulty is in knowing what movements and what postures will call forth certain kinds of breathing in what kind of people.'[5]

Classic Yoga texts similarly make it clear that breathing exercises were not taught before the student had undergone a long training in other aspects of Yoga, and then only under the personal guidance of an experienced guru, in a one-to-one situation.[6] (Since the masters of Yoga were so discrete about imparting their experience, it seems unsafe to assume that all present-day Yoga teaching has much connection with tradition.)

Taisen Deshimaru, writing about Zen and martial arts, says – amid some highly systematized advice on breathing! – that '*traditionally, the masters never taught it.*' (My italics)[7]

Many meditation techniques recommend observing the breath. But, as von Durckheim points out 'Anyone who has tried to observe his natural breath and consciously perform the act of breathing will be not a little astonished to see how his breath is suddenly and unnaturally disturbed by the very fact of its being put under observation.'[8]

Some Buddhist writers advise placing the attention on the movement of breath as it passes the tip of the nose on its way in and out. In that it tends to prevent useless or harmful intervention in what happens to the air after that, this seems a good idea for anyone who finds it difficult to leave well alone. Another Buddhist meditation suggests trying to observe the moment when in-breath gives way to out-breath and vice versa. Possibly the purpose of this meditation is the shock to received ideas when one finds that, when breathing is allowed to continue undisturbed, such a moment does not exist. (See **Chapter 11**.) This, for some, can be extremely disconcerting, even frightening. And once again, therefore, we come back to the idea that any experimentation of this kind calls for skilled guidance.

But if a skilled and experienced guide in these matters is rarely available in our society, must we therefore turn our backs on all such thoughts and questions that arise in us? If we see the dangers of lightly and hastily grasping at practices that are to be treated with respect (according to the repeated statements of those most likely to know) it is surely still open to us to consider the deep questions concerning our existence.

Through the clamour of advice and theory, there emerge clear voices which seem to come from some central point where authentic experiences touch each other. Sometimes in the language of poetry, sometimes in the terminology of vastly varying traditions, they remind us of the breath by which we live, of its freedom to come and go, of the fact that it is not ours to control but to receive. On the following pages are a few such utterances – no doubt others will occur to you. If any of them (from ancient sacred text to modern poetry) seem to speak to you, I hope you will listen to them patiently – quite possibly they have more to say.

The Master of the Universe said: 'I have created the four winds, so that each may breathe there where he finds himself...'
(Egyptian, *circa* 4000 B.C.)

And the Lord God formed man of the dust of the ground, and breathed into his nostrils the breath of life; and man became a living soul.
(Genesis 2:7)

Neither Being nor non-Being yet existed,
nor airy space, nor firmament beyond.
What stirred mightily? Where?...
Nothing yet distinguished night from day.
The One breathed of its own impulse, without breath.
Nothing else existed.
(Veda)

... a breath of life passed out from me
and by my own act I created living creatures.
(Isaiah 57:16)

Let me stretch out in the shade . . .
To turn my face to the lively breath of the west wind ...
(Hesiod, *circa* 700 B.C.)

It is by the earth in us that we know earth, and water by water, and by our air the divine air ...
(Empedocles, *circa* 493–*circa* 433 B.C.)

The wind blows where it wills, and you hear the sound of it, but you do not know whence it comes or whither it goes.
(John 3:8)

... breath, which we and the Greeks call 'air', life principle which penetrates the entire universe and is closely united with all...
(Pliny the Elder, 23–79)

The great flow of the ocean sets me moving, floating,
floating like algae on the surface of the water.
The celestial vault excites me and the powerful air stirs my spirit
and I fling myself in the dust.
I tremble with joy.
(Eskimo)

... Mine is this mysterious force of the invisible wind. I support the breath of all
that lives. I breathe in the verdure and in the flowers ... I am the force that lives
hidden in the winds ... as a man cannot act without breathing, so a fire cannot
burn but by my breath ... I impregnate all things, that they die not...
(Hildegarde von Bingen, 1098–1179)

The air is better being a living miracle as it now is than if it were crammed with
crowns and sceptres ... The freedom of Thy bounty hath deceived me. These
things were too near to be considered.
(Thomas Traherne, 1637–74)

... let the irresistible current of thy universal energy come like the impetuous
south wind of spring, let it come rushing over the vast field of the life of man, let
it bring the scent of many flowers and the murmurings of many woodlands...
(Rabindranath Tagore, 1861–1941)

My nose receives and transmits to my soul the wild scent of laurel,
the indefinable essence of the *boldo*...
(Pablo Neruda, 1904–73)

I lay me down under the coverlet of heaven,
And rest lightly on the pillows of the clouds...
Lie within my breast all night my love,
For I am the clouds, wind and the Breath of God.
(Clare Cameron)

If you think 'I breathe,' the 'I' is extra.
(Shunryu Suzuki, 1905–71 *Zen Mind, Beginner's Mind*)

1. Archbishop Anthony Bloom, *Living Prayer*, London, Darton, Longman and Todd, 1966, p. 87–8.
2. Chariton, Igumen of Valamo, *The Art of Prayer – an Orthodox Anthology*, London, Faber and Faber, 1966.
3. Hazrat Inayat Khan, *The Music of Life*, New York, Omega, 1983.
4. I. Gurdjieff, *Views from the Real World*, Dutton, 1973.
5. D. Ouspensky, *In Search of the Miraculous*, London, Routledge and Kegan Paul, 1950, p. 388.
6. Pantañjali, *How to know God – the Yoga aphorisms of Pantañjali*, transl. Swami Pravhavananda and C. Isherwood, Signet, 1969.
7. Taisen Deshimaru, *Zen et Arts Martiaux*, Paris, Seghers, 1977.
8. K. von Dürckheim, *The Japanese Cult of Tranquillity*, transl. E. O'Shiel, London, Rider, 1960, p. 34.

CHAPTER 13

THE CO-ORDINATING FACTOR

It is monstrous that the feet should direct the head.
Queen Elizabeth I of England

We have shared quite a lot by now, so no doubt you understand that from where I stand it does not appear that any approach which deals piecemeal with the human organism will ever get us very far. Everything in us is so interwoven, of such a marvellous complexity, that, if we take the piecemeal approach, while we try to correct one thing, another goes wrong. This is why I think most people would be a lot better off without those ubiquitous little articles telling us how to improve our posture, how to breathe, how to relax, and so forth. However much we know, we just can't take it all in at once; however much we fiddle about, we can't deal with everything at once. We can easily get ourselves into a hopeless muddle. If only there were some simple co-ordinating factor that would take care of some of the detail, leaving us free to think of other things. Well, there is.

The main co-ordinating factor is: the head. Extremely well co-ordinated people (some circus performers, for example) have always been aware of this – but probably not in a way that could be shared verbally. The facts were established scientifically more than seventy years ago, although their practical importance has not always been appreciated. Long before that, in the 1880s, the great pioneer F.M. Alexander, working empirically, discovered the essentials of co-ordination, and based his famous technique on them. (Chapter 34) His practical teaching continues to spread, but his books, on the whole, seem to be best understood by those who already know, from personal experience, what he meant. (Many recent writers seem to find the subject even more difficult to handle than Alexander did, so that much of the material most readily available in bookshops is misleading – but see 'Suggested reading', after Chapter 34.)

The present 'handbook', though owing much to my experience as an Alexander teacher since 1969, makes no attempt to describe the subtleties of the Alexander Technique in the hands of a good teacher. My more modest hope is that, by giving you such relevant facts and advice as I can write down in plain language, I may help you protect yourself from some of the misconceptions with which we have all been bombarded since childhood.

The head co-ordinates, not only because that is what we think with – but for all sorts of reasons, as I shall try to show. To understand why it is the principal co-ordinating factor, we shall need to go a little more deeply into questions of balance, with particular reference to the head and its relationship to the rest of the body. What about the *weight* of a head and its effect on the rest? Heads vary in size – and of course children's heads are larger in proportion to their bodies – but even in adult life, your head represents a considerable weight, sitting on top there. It really is quite a balancing feat we are performing all day long, when you come to think of it! The human body when vertical, whether still or in movement, is essentially an unstable structure, in that its mass tapers to a base formed by its little feet. It stands to reason that the placing of a large, mobile weight – the head – at the top of this structure has an important influence on the balance of the whole.

For some reason it often happens that when I try to discuss questions of balance with people, I meet with a certain reluctance: 'I am not mechanically minded ... I never studied physics'. But there are certain things you can't help knowing; and you act upon this knowledge every day. Suppose I am holding the lamps in fig. 20; you certainly know that lamp b) is going to fall if I let go of it, and that lamp a) will probably come back, wobble a bit and finally stand on its base. The difference? Most of the weight in b) is already tending to fall *outside* the base, whereas in a) most of the weight is tending to fall *within* the base. Bear in mind that people are just as much subject to gravity as lamps are – but we have more choice about how we react. To help you to focus your attention on what you certainly know already, here are a few simple experiments worth making.

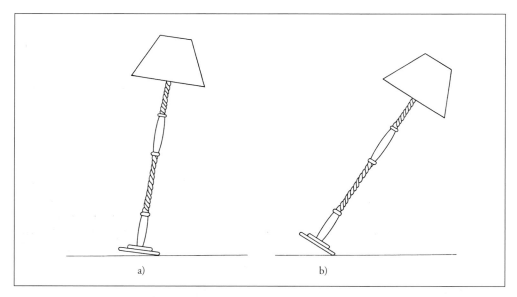

a)   b)

— *Fig. 20* —

You can't help knowing that lamp b) will certainly fall, whereas lamp a) may be all right.

86

❏ *Experiment 1*

Make a tower of children's bricks, six of the smallest bricks at the bottom, an equal height of bigger bricks on top of them. Then another small one and, lastly, put one of the biggest bricks on top of your tower. See how carefully you have to place it, to avoid toppling the lot! Of course, this is very different from a human body, but I think it helps to highlight some questions of balance that we deal with all the time without realizing it (fig. 21).

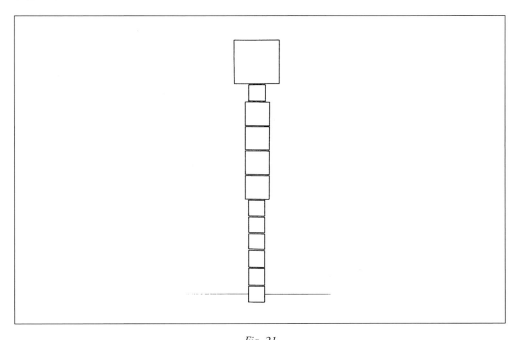

— *Fig. 21* —

See how carefully you have to place the top brick.

❏ *Experiment 2*

If you can do so with your heels on the ground, go into a deep squat. (If you can't do this easily, never mind, just stand in front of a low sofa with your back to it, as if you were thinking of sitting on it. Then get as near to a squat as you comfortably can *without lifting your heels*.) Now, see if you can look up at the ceiling, moving only your head. How did you get on? Did you topple backwards and end up sitting on the floor (or sofa)? If you kept your balance, how did you manage it? Did you

a) hold on to something?

b) hold yourself in place by an increased effort in your legs and feet?

c) move your arms forwards?

d) fold at the waist?

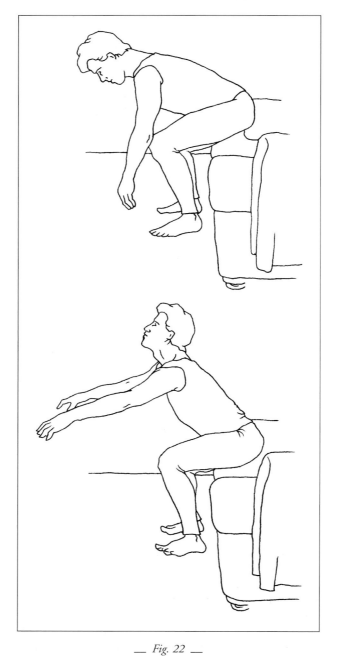

— *Fig. 22* —

Attempt at squatting: head influences balance.

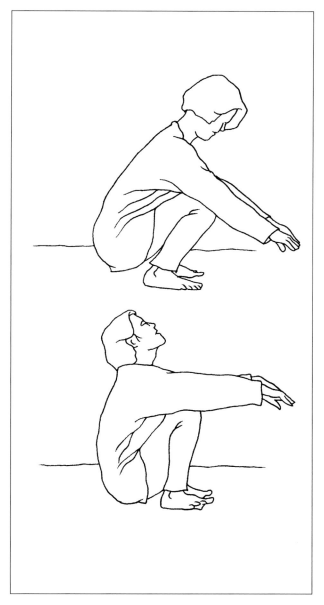

— *Fig. 23* —

Here, a precarious squat is easily upset when the head attitude
changes. (Inadequate lateral thigh rotation adds to the difficulty –
see Chapter 21.)

In your squat you were just balanced, with some weight (your seat) behind your base (your feet) while probably your head and upper body were a bit forward to compensate. When you moved an important weight (your head) backwards, you created a balance problem. Reactions a) and b) are attempts to solve that problem by making increased muscular efforts to stay where you are; c) and d) are attempts to solve the balance problem by putting extra weight forward to compensate for the backward displacement of the weight of the head. Whatever happened, I think you will have noticed that *the shifting of the head's weight had an effect on your balance and imposed some sort of compensatory behaviour on you* (figs. 22, 23).

I have purposely taken a fairly extreme example. But in fact, whether you notice it or not, the placing of the head always makes some difference to the rest of you. In one sense this is simply mechanical, just like the tower of bricks. But changes in the placing of the head also bring about changes in muscular behaviour.[1] This is normal and natural. Dancers and acrobats have an awareness of the process (even if they don't give it a name). Gray's *Anatomy* makes a passing reference to it[2] – without underlining the enormous practical importance it has for us all. (The purpose of Gray's is to give facts, not to place them in order of importance.) If you experiment as suggested, you will realize that you have a measure of choice in the way in which balance is achieved and maintained.

Of course, none of this means that we should maintain a fixed position of the head – quite the contrary, as we shall see. Tiny head movements can cause significant changes elsewhere in the body, so it is interesting to see how they work. While you are reading the description in the next chapter, please *don't try to feel* what I am explaining. Some of the mechanisms are so delicate that there is almost no sensation involved, therefore to try to feel them could create confusion. It is better just to read and understand. As we proceed, I shall suggest little experiments you can make if you want to test my explanations.

---

1. R. Magnus, 'Some results of studies in the physiology of posture' (Cameron Prize Lectures), *Lancet*, Sept. 11, 1926, discussing animal movements: 'It is possible, by giving to the head different positions, to change the distribution of tone in the whole body musculature...'
2. Gray's *Anatomy*, p. 1152 (Neurology).

CHAPTER 14

HEAD MOVEMENTS:
(1) LOOKING UP AND DOWN, NODDING

> Human beings have a specific structure – like any other
> species – and can grow only in terms of this structure.
> Freedom does not mean freedom from all guiding prin-
> ciples. It means freedom to grow according to the laws of
> human existence. It means obedience to the laws that gov-
> ern optimal human development.
>
> Erich Fromm *To Have or To Be*

> ... it is essential, when pinching policemen's helmets, to
> give a forward shove before applying the upward lift.
> Otherwise, the subject's chin catches in the strap ... There
> is a right way and a wrong way...
>
> P. G. Wodehouse *The Code of the Woosters*

In Chapter 4, we talked about the joint between the head and the top of the spine, and about the common mistake of imagining it to be somewhere at the back of the neck. In fig. 24 you will notice two little knobs (*occipital condyles*) which form part of the base of the skull. They are like tiny rockers and they sit in a pair of small cups (the superior articular surfaces of the *atlas* or first cervical vertebra) – at the very top of your spine. Note how high this is and how far forward. Picture this joint between your ears (scarcely below the level of the ear-holes) and you won't go far wrong.

The two 'cups' are shaped into the upper surface of the atlas vertebra in such a way that the 'rockers' can't slip out, however freely we allow them to move. Ligaments hold them in place, and of course there is cushioning and lubrication. The condyles can rock within their 'cups', slipping backwards and forwards to produce a small nodding movement of the head, as when you are quietly agreeing with someone. Kapandji gives the range of this movement as fifteen degrees.[1] Many people, however, place unconscious limits on this movement in themselves, replacing it by movements of the whole neck – an error so common that it has even led to some confusion in terminology.[2]

There is also at this level a very slight lateral tilting movement of which the total range is three degrees, according to Kapandji.[3] What we usually think of as 'tilting the head' is a movement carried out principally in the neck. *Turning* the head also occurs elsewhere. (It is discussed in Chapter 16.)

The head-atlas joint has a characteristic that is of immense practical importance to

91

us. In order to understand it we shall compare it with another joint: the elbow. As you read, I invite you to make some little experiments.

❏ *Experiment 1*

(a) Standing or sitting with the whole arm straight at shoulder height, bend the arm at the elbow. You have contracted flexor muscles attached to the inside of your arm above and below the elbow; this pulled your forearm towards your upper arm.

(b) Now straighten your arm again. You have contracted extensor muscles attached to the back of your arm above and below the elbow. You have released the flexors accordingly, but that release alone would not have straightened your arm when it was in that position. The movement called for the contraction of the extensors – let us say an *active use of the joint*, by which I mean that it depends on muscular contraction.

❏ *Experiment 2*

(a) Start with the arm hanging normally from the shoulder. Leaving the upper arm where it is, bend the elbow. Again you have contracted flexors, as you did in 1(a). Clearly, this too, is *active*.

(b) Keep your elbow in its bent position for a few seconds. You are maintaining a flexor contraction – so obviously this also is *active*.

(c) Simply let your forearm drop. Your arm has *straightened because your flexors are no longer opposing the force of gravity.* This time you didn't need to use your extensors, did you? You only needed to stop holding your elbow bent.

In Experiment 1, you contracted flexors and extensors in turn, i.e. you *did* both bending and straightening. In Experiment 2(c), you didn't need to *do* the straightening; gravity could do it for you. Let us call this a *passive use* of the joint. Obvious? Yes, indeed. An obvious example of the difference between *doing* and *allowing to happen*. A consideration of the obvious can often help us to understand things that are less immediately apparent.

Most joints can be used actively or passively, according to circumstances. *But the head-atlas joint is unique. In one direction, effectively the head can only move passively* – as your arm moved in Experiment 2(c). We shall see why.

❏ *Experiment 3*

If you get on hands and knees, pretending to be a four-footed animal, you will realize that if you want to have a good look at your surroundings you will lift your face by pulling the back of your head towards your back. (Several muscles can participate in this action, mostly by pulling the head towards the spine, while the large and powerful pair called *trapezius* can also pull it towards the shoulders.) For the sake of brevity I shall call this action *pulling the head backwards*. This seems to me the simplest way of describing this movement. It is clear to us in the all-fours position. In the upright position we might think of it as 'lifting the face'. The fact remains, however, that the muscular action is that of pulling the head towards your back.

Still considering *only* the movements at the head-atlas joint, the backwards move-ment of the head is accomplished most smoothly if you let your eyes lead the way. The head moves very naturally to make it easy for you to look where you want to look. When this is finished with, when you have done with looking up, you won't need to use muscle power to return your head to its original 'neutral' position: *gravity does it for you, once you stop holding your head backwards* – just as it did for your arm in Experiment 2(c). *The passive use of the joint is the only way of making the genuine return to neutral.*

Of course, the head, like the arm, can be released at different speeds – but do not try to drop it abruptly. *It is really a matter of where you want to look.* So, when you simply de-cide that you no longer need to pull or hold your head backwards, it does not follow that everything collapses! No, your head just returns naturally to 'neutral', while the intricate network of stretch reflexes continues to function for your protection.

It is of course possible to let your *neck* drop, too, like an animal that wants to crop the grass. This is not the movement we are discussing at the moment, but many people confuse the two – which makes the next experiment important.

❏ *Experiment 4*

I suggest you try the two, to appreciate the difference between
(a) dropping your *head* and
(b) dropping your *neck*.
At the base of the neck you can feel two knobs (the spines of the seventh cervical and first thoracic vertebrae). From this region, where neck and back meet, your neck can drop quite a lot, if you so choose.

Whether you drop the neck or keep it more or less continuous with the back, you can pull the head backwards (as I have described) and let it drop forward again. These are smaller movements and the head is moving from its joint between the ears – a long way away from the meeting-place of neck and back.

I stress this point because many people are not aware of this distinction between head and neck. Of course you can move them together or separately – it is up to you. But if you don't know that the choice exists, you may use head and neck as if they were soldered together. Many people do so – and many problems are caused by this confusion of head and neck.

Let us follow this line of thought a bit further. Suppose I am in my kitchen and I want to look up at a high shelf. As I have said, attached to the back of my head are several pairs of muscles which can be brought into action to pull my head towards my spine (and, in the case of trapezius, towards my shoulder-blades). This, of course, tilts my head: the back of it is pulled down and the face is therefore upwards. Of course I can use my muscles to do this any time I like – that is what they are for. The important point is that when I want to look straight forward again, gravity will still do the job, just as it did when I was on all fours. This is because *the centre of gravity of the head is slightly in front of the head-atlas joint, so the head will always drop gently into 'neutral' when I am not holding it some-where else.*

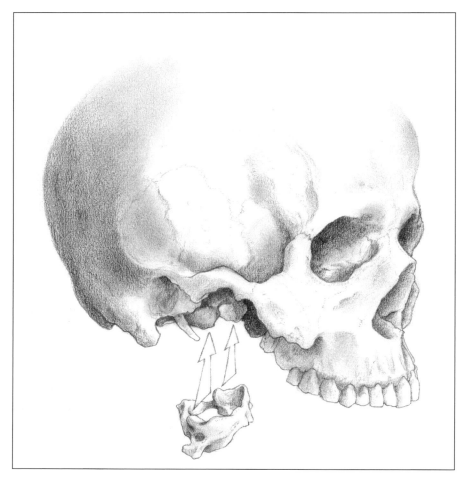

— *Fig. 24* —
Skull showing condyles

We saw (**in Chapter 6**) how muscles can co-operate by opposing each other; we take this for granted, and often assume we can *do* one action, and then reverse it by *doing* the opposite. *This is a dangerous assumption, because there is no effective antagonist to all the muscular forces capable of pulling the head backwards.*[4] In fact, none is needed: the weight of the head provides the necessary opposition.[5] Fig. 25 shows the principle in action.
W = weight; P = power; F = fulcrum – this is where the joint is.

Here is another little experiment which may make all this clearer to you. As with all my suggested experiments, if it doesn't seem to clarify things for you immediately, please do not persist. There are other, less direct ways of arriving at the same understanding.

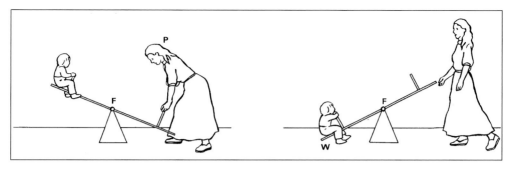

Because of the opposing weight of the child, the lighter end of the see-saw rises when the woman stops holding it down.

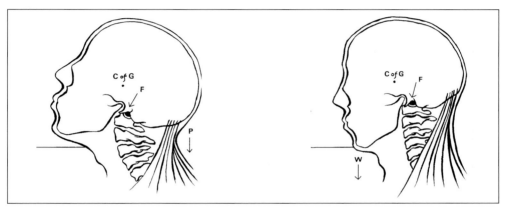

Because of the opposing weight of the heavier front of the head, the lighter back of the head rises when the muscles stop holding it down.

___ *Fig. 25* ___

The weight of the head provides opposition to muscles that pull the head backwards. (For important implications, see Chapter 17.)

❏ *Experiment 5*

(You can try this experiment for yourself, three or four times only – there is no point in doing more. On no account do it to anyone else – it would be easy to do them harm, however gentle you are.)

Sit close to a table (dining height, not a low coffee-table) and put your elbows on the table. With your middle fingers, gently find the little dent just behind the lobes of your ears (between the jaw and the skull). Leaving your fingers where they are, and with your mouth closed, put the tips of your thumbs under your chin. Provided your head joint is 'in neutral', a very gentle push upwards with your thumbs (elbows still on the table) will be enough to tilt your face upwards just a bit, i.e. to tip your whole head slightly backwards without you *pulling* it towards your back. (If this doesn't seem to work for you, *don't* increase the thumb pressure and *don't* use muscle power to move your head. Either would be counter-productive.)

When you stop pushing with your thumbs, you will probably find that your head will tip gently forward towards its original position, touching your thumbs again. This is what will happen if the joint continues to be 'in neutral'. Of course, if you prefer, instead of letting the head tip forward by its own weight, you can intervene so as to hold your head in its tipped-back position. *The whole point is to notice that the choice is yours.* Note that the head can be made to travel further backwards than its joint allows for, if you also bend the neck backwards. If you do this, the experiment will not be valid, as the movement will no longer be purely a head movement.

The reason I have devoted so much explanation to the head-atlas joint is that very few people realize where it is and how it functions. So, although most people can usually move their heads or hold them still, they are quite unaware of the third possibility, which I call the *neutral* state of the joint, in which it is simply available for movement. Although you may not necessarily choose to take up the movement option at any given moment, this neutral state, when it exists, creates conditions that are decidedly advantageous for the rest of the body.

Let me explain how this works. As we have seen, many muscles can participate in pulling the head backwards in this joint[6]; there are only two pairs of small muscles capable of acting in the opposite sense[7] and *they are not powerful enough to compete with the combined muscular forces concerned in the backward pull.* These two pairs co-operate with other deep muscles (those concerned in sideways, backwards, and rotational pulls on the head[8]) to make small adjustments when we are standing, sitting, moving around. Here, at the core, so to speak, of everything that moves the head, are tiny muscles which – when not being overruled by stronger forces – are continuously at work to balance the head and to place it in the most advantageous position for the balance of the whole body. The ideal balance of the head is, of course, something constantly changing according to what actions the rest of the body is called upon to perform. (**More about the implications in Chapters 15–17.**) These deep muscles will always take care of head balance provided they are allowed to do so.

❏ *Experiment 6*

Place the fingers and thumb of one hand together in a bunch and on the tips balance a large beach ball or similar object. Walk or dance about the room, noticing how your fingers co-operate with each other by tiny movements to keep the ball in balance. This will give a rough working idea of the continuous reflex activity of the muscles immediately surrounding the head-atlas joint.

The continuous interplay of these muscles is brought about by stretch reflexes, by the muscles' reaction to gravity and to each other. It is a subtle and delicate reflex system which leaves no room for well-meant interference. You should not try to control it or even to feel it. All it requires is that you don't overrule it unnecessarily.

I seem to hear you ask: 'But how am I to be sure that I'm not overruling it?' A good question, which I shall attempt to answer by another suggested experiment.

❏ *Experiment 7*

Do this just where you are and as you are, *without moving.*
(a) Imagine that someone you don't much like wants to move your head and you are certainly not going to let them do so.
(b) Now pretend to yourself that the person whose touch you like best in all the world wants to move your head very gently and you don't mind in the least!

I am sure you were confident in both cases that your head was prepared to react as you required it to in these imagined situations. You probably don't have any clear idea of what the difference was – that doesn't matter. All that really matters to you is that your muscles were obedient, as usual. In 7(a) I expect the muscles around the joint contracted all at once to lock the head to the atlas. (Probably quite a few other muscles got in on the act as well.) In 7(b) most likely the muscles in question calmed down and returned to their job of gently adapting to circumstances. So you see, you have more control than you feel as though you have. Quite often things change in a moment in response to your wishes!

If this seems like a fairy tale, let me ask you: how on earth do you so much as take a sip of water or a mouthful of food? The description of swallowing takes practically a whole page in Gray's *Anatomy*, yet you can do it just like that![9] And 'just like that' you have just had an effect on the availability of your head to the action of your own reflexes – no need to work it out, still less to check up to see if your requests are being carried out.

Talking of fairy tales, there is one about a man who was given three wishes. He wasted two of them by wishing absent-mindedly for things he didn't really want, with such disastrous results that the only solution was... to use the third wish to wish that none of it had ever happened! If we are to avoid wishing for muscular efforts that only cancel each other out, we need to do some clear thinking about what we really wish to happen.

It must be said that for some people the mechanisms described don't seem to respond easily to a simple wish, even though the person has understood intellectually what is involved. When that is the case, there is often a simple explanation; specific disease or injury being ruled out, the problem is usually rooted in habits and misunderstandings. It often turns out that in the past such a person has given the musculature so many contradictory instructions that the concept of a neutral state becomes elusive in the extreme.

In such a case, it is reasonable to look for help. There is no magic wand that will enable one to function better without learning to make some changes. Alexander teachers are people who have been trained specifically to guide people through this kind of difficulty. It can be important to seek the advice of a qualified teacher who actually sees and knows you. This book is not a set of DIY instructions.

However, with appropriate information, we can often avoid complicating our problems: at least, when we feel the need to compensate for difficulties whose real nature remains unclear, we can pause for thought. And this is already something, for *only that pause will allow any solution to be effective.* (See Chapter 10.) In the next two chapters, still putting together the jigsaw puzzle that is our body-image, let us look further into head movements.

---

1. I.A. Kapandji, *The Physiology of the Joints*, Edinburgh, Churchill Livingstone, 1974, vol. 3, p. 184.
2. Some examples:
    a) W. Platzer, *Color Atlas and Textbook of Human Anatomy, vol.1, Locomotor System*, New York, Thieme, 4th English edition, 1992, p. 322:
    'Bilateral contraction (of the sternocleidomastoid) lifts the head.'
    It is not clear what is meant here. In the erect posture, the sternocleidomastoids obviously cannot 'lift the head'. When the body is supine, however, and depending on the action of other muscles (including abdominals) they can participate in lifting the head clear of the surface on which it is lying.
    b) F.P. Kendall and E.K. McCreary, *Muscles – Testing and function*, Baltimore, Williams and Wilkins, 3rd edition, 1983, p. 260:
    'In an habitually faulty position with *forward head* (my italics) the sternocleidomastoid muscles remain in a shortened position, and tend to develop shortness.'
    This is certainly true, but it needs to be said that it is really the *neck* that is forward; the *head*, although 'forward' in space, i.e. relative to the trunk, is usually tilted backwards and down, relative to the cervical spine, in an attempt to counteract imbalance, and so that the eyes can look ahead – as in the Kendall illustration on p. 300.
    c) J.V. Basmajian, *Primary Anatomy*, Baltimore, Williams and Wilkins, 7th edition, 1976, p. 128:
    'When right and left sternomastoids contract simultaneously the head and neck are flexed.'
    Similarly vague descriptions are to be found wherever authors treat the head and neck as though the existence of the atlanto-occipital joint were of purely theoretical interest. They seem to reflect general confusion as to the practicalities underlying problems in this area. For greater clarity concerning the action of the sternocleidomastoids, see: T.D.M. Roberts, *Understanding Balance*, London, Chapman and Hall, 1995, p. 103.
3. Kapandji, *op. cit.*, p. 184.
4. The role of the muscles *longus capitis* and *rectus capitis anterior* is discussed later in this chapter.
5. Kapandji, *op. cit.* p. 216, describes this as:
    'a lever system ... the fulcrum lies at the level of the occipital condyles ... force is produced by the weight of the head applied through its centre of gravity near the *sella turcica*; posterior neck muscles ... counterbalance the weight of the head...'
6. In addition to the suboccipital muscles *rectus capitis posterior major and minor and obliquus capitis superior*, we can list *longissimus capitis, semispinalis capitis, splenius capitis, trapezius* (see Chapter 33, notes 5 and 6) and *sternocleidomastoid* (see note 2b above).
7. *longus capitis, rectus capitis anterior*.
8. *rectus capitis lateralis, and the suboccipital group of muscles*.
9. Gray's *Anatomy*, pp. 1249–50 (Splanchology).

CHAPTER 15

HEAD MOVEMENTS:
(2) THE JAW AND ITS INFLUENCE

> Any animal, and man especially, is a highly integrated
> structure, all the parts of which must change together as
> his behaviour changes. The evolution of the hand, of the
> eyes, of the feet, the teeth, the whole human frame, made
> a mosaic of special gifts.
>
> J. Bronowski *The Ascent of Man*

It can be surprising to find that a major obstacle to good head balance often arises from the way the lower jaw is used. Whether eating, speaking, singing, or merely swallowing saliva, people quite often acquire habits that work against the free poise of the head that is so essential to all efficient use of our mechanisms. We can distinguish between habits due to misunderstandings about jaw functioning, and habits due to the emotions, probably rooted in our evolutionary history.

Let's look first at the misunderstandings, which in my experience are principally concerned with opening the mouth. I often ask people to represent, by means of sketches or hand movements, what they think happens when the mouth is opened. These illustrations generally fall into three categories:
a) the whole lower jaw is shown descending vertically – coming apart from its moorings, one might say;
b) something like the 'shadow pictures' one used to make as a child, of a crocodile opening its mouth, raising the upper jaw;
c) something like an upside-down box, with the lid dangling by the hinge.

The first of these illustrations is a clear impossibility. As soon as you think about it, you realize that the lower jaw must be attached to something above – in fact, to the skull – and attached further back than the chin, since the chin does drop. Indeed, people whose mental picture corresponds to a) are usually frank about admitting they 'don't quite know how it does that' – and are quite relieved to learn that in fact it doesn't. Illustrations b) and c) are possible, but have disadvantages. The people who choose the 'crocodile' option are usually quick to see that it necessarily implies pulling the head backwards, in view of the fact that the upper jaw forms part of the skull. The snag with the 'up-turned box' choice is a little more difficult to appreciate, because it is just possible to use the lower jaw like this and not move the head – but in fact this is uncomfortable, particularly for the larynx, so in this case too, you would almost certainly end up by pulling your head backwards.

Really, the lower jaw is supposed to slide forwards as the chin drops. Of course, the chin eventually moves nearer to the neck again – since any joint movement results in an arc – but by then, thanks to the forward component, the discomfort has been avoided. In this way, the mouth can open fairly wide without inconvenience, and without disturbing the head balance. There are muscles for moving the jaw forward and down (for opening the mouth) and backward and up (for bringing the teeth together). The resting position is between the two, with a little space between the upper and lower teeth, even when the lips are together. In view of gravity, when one is vertical a small amount of muscle activity is needed to keep the mouth from falling open when we don't want it to. Opening it depends largely on release of these muscles – and should not really be much work. (As you know, it's often easy enough when you fall asleep in a train.)

Unfortunately, understanding all this doesn't always prevent the jaw from being held too tightly to move properly. Jaw muscles are very powerful and we often use much more of their power than is appropriate to what we are doing. I think evolution must have something to do with this. On land or in the sea, for creatures that prey on others, good jaw muscles are a requirement – muscles quick to snap, strong enough to hold on when your dinner is making frantic efforts to escape. Surely these muscles express the very essence of the creature's determination to survive. In the changed circumstances of human existence, we often express determination by clenching our teeth; it can become a habit to use all that power for nothing more strenuous than stopping our mouths from gaping open!

❏ *Experiment 1*

Try saying, with as much vehemence as you can put into it, something like 'I swear I am going to finish this job tonight if it kills me!' – I think you will see what I mean. Ask yourself if you recognize this as something you do when confronting a difficulty.

❏ *Experiment 2*

Pretend to be a baby sucking: without pulling your head backwards, place the tip of your little finger lightly against your lips. Reach for it with lips and tongue, draw it into your mouth and suck rhythmically and vigorously, as if really expecting to get some nourishment out of it. Watch your profile in the mirror: does your jaw move forwards and backwards as you suck, from a point just in front of your ears? N.B. Don't use your thumb for this: the idea is to evoke memories of *sucking for sustenance* (not to be confused with thumb sucking for comfort, which may well be a later memory).

❏ *Experiment 3*

As you sit reading this, without changing anything, ask yourself whether your teeth are touching each other, or whether there is a little space between them. Then ask yourself what your tongue is doing. Is it moving a lot in your mouth? Is it resting quietly and if so, where?

❏ *Experiment 4*

Sometimes, when you need to swallow saliva, notice how you do so. Do you let your jaw move forward like a baby's? If your teeth meet, do they touch lightly, or do you clench them? Most important: do you pull your head backwards? (If so, think how many times a day it must be happening!) Perhaps you could pause occasionally for a second before swallowing, with the intention of leaving your head free when you do so.

A little experimentation on these lines could help you to ensure that your jaw does not put the free balance of your head at unnecessary risk.

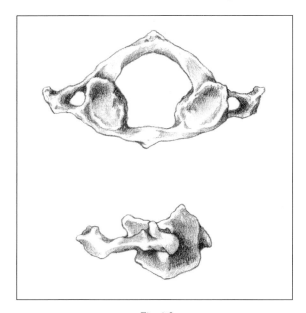

— *Fig. 26* —

Atlas from above and in profile

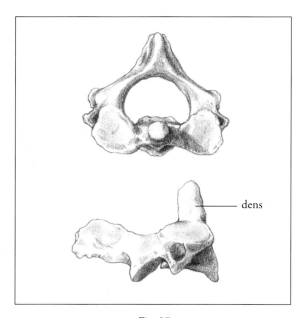

— *Fig. 27* —

Axis from above and in profile

CHAPTER 16

HEAD MOVEMENTS:
(3) TURNING THE HEAD

> When the postural development of the individual is such as to place at the disposal of the forebrain a perfectly poised apparatus, the conscious and subconscious aspects of movement are happily integrated.
>
> Raymond A. Dart *The postural aspect of malocclusion*

Whereas the nodding movement occurs when the head moves on the first vertebra, the head turning movements occur between the first and second vertebrae. The first vertebra is called the *atlas* (fig. 26) because the head rests on it; the second, on which turning occurs, is called the *axis* (fig. 27). The top of the axis forms a peg which fits into the front part of the hole in the atlas, being kept in place by a ligament; the shape of the joint surfaces allows the atlas to swivel around the peg of the axis. (The peg looks rather like a tooth and is known as the *dens* of the axis.) It is apparent from the shape of the bones that the relationship of the head to the atlas does not allow for turning: in the turning movement, head and atlas go together.

A number of muscles are involved in turning the head. Most of them, besides turning the head, tend to tilt it backwards – which is all very well if you want to look sideways and upwards. But the backward tendency can become inconvenient if what you want to see is at eye level or below. For instance, you may need to watch your hands doing all sorts of things, from washing dishes to playing the piano; or to look in your wing mirror at cars coming up in the fast lane. In such cases, you may end up doing awkward compensatory movements unless you observe certain precautions.

What precautions? First, allow the head's weight its freedom, thus restoring the head-atlas joint to its 'neutral condition'. (**Chapter 14**) This minimizes pressure on the atlas-axis joint, besides being advantageous for the muscles concerned. Then seek the object you want to see ... *with the eye that is further away from the object.*

I know this sounds strange, but there are good reasons for it. The neurological relationship between eye movements and head movements is complex, but we can draw some simple conclusions, of which one of the most useful is this: if you want your head to turn to the left easily and smoothly, ask your right eye to look briefly towards the point of your left shoulder before going on to look elsewhere – and vice versa.[1] This simple procedure has several advantages:

a) Neck mechanisms are protected from unnecessary wear and tear. (Even if you want to look up with a sideways tilt of the head, you are much less likely to hurt yourself if you start the movement as suggested.)
b) If it is necessary to look further than a movement at the atlas-axis joint can accomplish unaided, mechanisms lower down in the neck and in the thorax will play their part smoothly if the movement has been begun correctly.
c) You will see better this way than you will if your head turning is abrupt and ill coordinated.

Let me suggest some experiments here. Again, let me stress that these are not exercises but what I may call explorations. Intellectual understanding is important in its way, but only when you have 'been there' will your understanding come progressively to belong to you. So I hope you will make experiments – remembering that a true experiment does not always turn out as you expect!

❏ *Experiment 1*

On all fours, head dropped, neck not dropped (see **Chapter 14**) and with your right eye shut: look at your right hand with your left eye; then look at the floor further still to the right, allowing your head to turn as necessary. Then close your left eye, and look with your right eye at your left hand and further. Try the same thing with both eyes open but still with the idea 'further eye leads'. Compare this with what happens when you lead with the near eye; true, the head doesn't have to turn as far to see the same thing – but does the movement have the same smooth quality?

❏ *Experiment 2*

In a fairly large room, or out of doors, walk briskly to a pre-decided point, turn without stopping and walk briskly back. For interesting results, this should be done without any hesitation at the turn, walking at the same speed throughout. Do this in two ways:
a) the head maintains absolutely the same relationship to the shoulders, the eyes looking straight ahead – like a tin soldier;
b) the further eye tries to look across the shoulder to see the way you expect to go when you turn. (Yes, I know your nose is in the way, but that doesn't matter when both eyes are open.) The head, of course, is allowed to go with the eye movement. Naturally, the other eye leads the head to a forward-looking position after the turn has been accomplished. Do left and right turns and compare them. Is it easier to turn to the left or to the right? Could the easier side teach the other how easy it really is?

Important practical applications for road safety

I assure you that there are plenty of painful and distracting 'stiff necks' that have absolutely nothing to do with the draughty car windows that are usually blamed for them. What is more, it is all too easy, particularly if the traffic is making you a bit nervous or impatient, to make a jerky head-turning movement that can even cause you to 'see stars' for a moment ... a moment in which an accident could happen.

I know you don't want to try out new things in the middle of busy traffic. But when you have prepared by experimenting at home, try reminding yourself of this advice when looking to see if it is safe to emerge from a parking place. I expect you will find it so natural that soon you will be doing it also when preparing to overtake.

Think about all this sometimes, casually, as you walk about your home. Let the further eye lead your head, and your head lead your body towards the next thing you want to do. One advantage is the gradual realization that the head need not be held fixed just because you are doing something that does not require continuous movement. There are times when we need to look mostly straight ahead – driving on a motorway, for example, or watching the screen of a computer, as I am now. At such times it is not necessary to keep moving the head to prove that it is not fixed: it is quite possible just to leave it in a neutral state, temporarily immobile but still available for movement. Some people feel themselves getting stiff whenever they are doing something that does not involve much movement. They need to recognize that it is perfectly possible to be fairly still without using muscle to fix the parts concerned. Experiment 7 in Chapter 14 can be adapted to suit head turning movements. The thought in this case becomes 'I wouldn't mind if someone gently nodded my head and then turned it a bit.' This leads to a realization that when the head is available for passive movement in this way, it is also available for small movements initiated by our own eyes. Many people don't realize how often they move like toy soldiers, as if the head were soldered to the body. They feel so much better once a little thought has paved the way for other, pleasanter possibilities.

Before we leave this subject, *a word of warning* against exercises that involve 'rolling the head' (fig. 28). This is exercise for the sake of exercise – with a vague idea of doing oneself good. Some people imagine that it frees the neck: I can only assure them that they are seriously mistaken. Nobody would think of moving the head this way in real life and I do not think it does any good to anyone. Natural movements are purposeful. The usual purpose in moving one's head is to see something – but what can anyone expect to see while rolling the head about? Such exercises are very far removed from any idea of collecting visual information, and tend to confuse the co-ordination. (If you like dancing in discos, I'd like to suggest that you may find it even more enjoyable when the head is freely balanced than when it is rolling in all directions – try it, you might start a fashion.)

I know that for people subject to 'stiff necks' due to habits of misuse, these exercises may bring an illusion of relief, whereas in fact they run counter to the possibility of improved use. That is because they take no account of all the intricate interplay of muscles by which nature permits your gaze to travel where you want it to. If you move your head simply and naturally, by letting it follow your eye movements, you will not need such exercises and will be better without them. An essential requirement of good muscular co-ordination is to let interest in what you are looking at (or looking for) guide your head movements, as it did when you were little (fig. 29).

1. R.A. Dart, *The Attainment of Poise* (1947) reprinted in Dart, *Skill and Poise*, London, STAT Books, 1996, p. 141: '... closure of one eye facilitates rotation of the head and the whole body towards the temporarily blind side.'

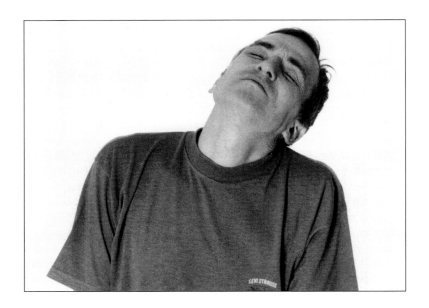

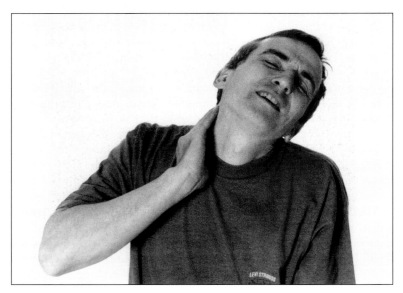

— *Fig. 28* —
Head-rolling: an exercise better avoided

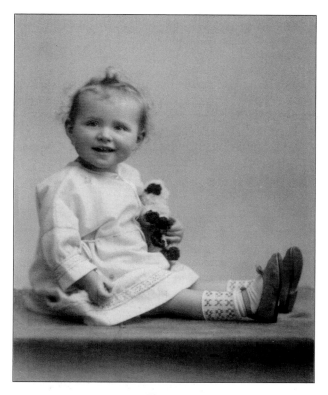

— Fig. 29 —

Let your interest in what you are looking at guide your head movements, as it did when you were a young child.

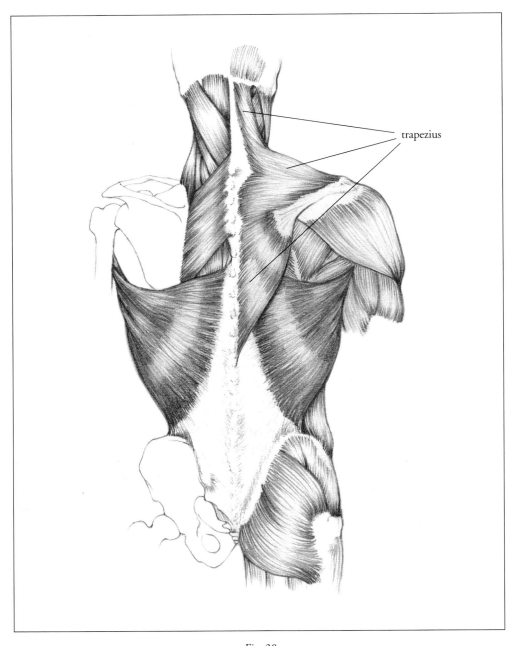

trapezius

— Fig. 30 —
Back muscles: first layer (right); second layer (left)

CHAPTER 17

HOW THE HEAD AFFECTS THE FRAMEWORK

Knowledge is not a loose-leaf notebook of facts. Above all,
it is a responsibility for the integrity of what we are.

J. Bronowski *The Ascent of Man*

In bipedal man, the relationship of the head to the erect
body is of primary importance.

Raymond A. Dart *Voluntary musculature in the human
body: the double spiral arrangement*

... what is the principle of the arch? You can call it, if you
like, an affront to gravitation; you would be more correct
if you call it an appeal to gravitation. The principle asserts
that by combining separate stones of a particular shape in
a particular way, we can ensure that their very tendency to
fall shall prevent them from falling.

G. K. Chesterton *Essays*

At an early foetal stage, the head is much the biggest part of us. When we are small children, it is still very big in proportion to the rest – a weight to be reckoned with. By the time we are old enough to think about these things, our bodies have grown quite a lot bigger than our heads. Then we tend to think of the head as the place where we think, the body as the 'physical' part of us, forgetting something that by instinct we took for granted when we were very small: the important influence that the head, considered purely as a *weight*, has on the way all the rest of us functions.

When you experimented with squatting and moving the head (**Chapter 13**) you saw how easily a small movement of the head could upset or help your balance. Now I should like to explain some of the more far-reaching effects the head can have on the framework as a whole.

We have already talked about the big muscle systems supporting the body in its upright posture. (**Chapter 8**) I likened these systems to ropes holding up a tent: in essence they are similar, but of course a lot more complicated. Figs. 30–32 show several layers of back muscles: you can see that, viewed as a system, all that musculature can hardly be considered without reference to all the attachments to the back of the head.

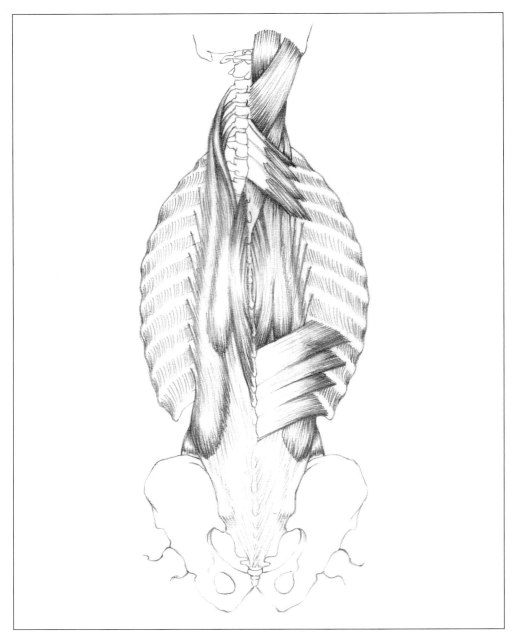

— *Fig. 31* —
Back muscles: third layer (right); fourth layer (left)

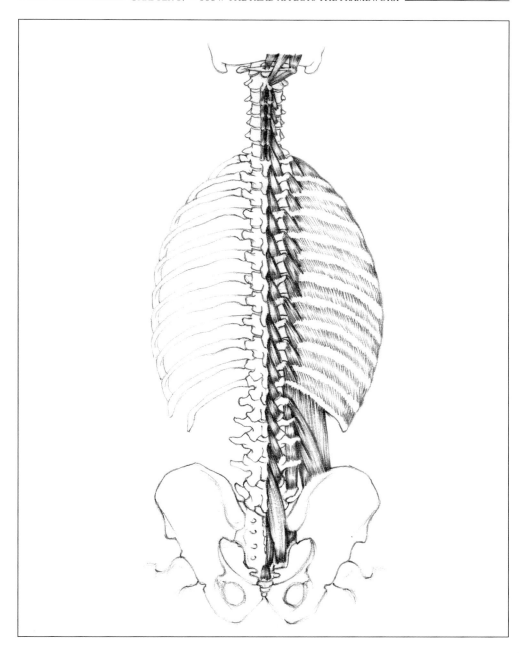

_ *Fig. 32* _
Back muscles: deepest layer

I have pointed out that the top of the spine is not only higher up but also further forward than many people realize; so that the head is better supported than you may have thought. (**Chapter 4**) However, don't forget that the heavier part of the head is in front of the head-atlas joint. (**Chapter 14**) When we considered the head, balanced on the atlas, we noticed a tendency for the face to drop a bit, so that naturally the back of the head rises. (Think of a see-saw or an old-fashioned pair of scales.) Now I want to draw your attention to the fact that when the back of the head rises, it tends to take up slack in the vertical muscles of the back, as you would expect. In this way, the weight of the head, as it drops slightly forward in its joint, can exert a gentle stretch on the whole vertical system of back muscles, thus rendering them more tonic, more ready for the demands we may be about to make on them. In some ways it's like a pulley system.

This is the stretch reflex at work again. (**Chapter 7**) As we know, muscles contract when they are stretched. Let us not forget, however, that muscles can pull in either direction, according to what movements you decide on. If what you want is for the heavier front of the head to stay dropped so that the back part can continue to rise, that is what will occur. (I repeat, the *head* drops forward, not the neck!) The head will keep the *top* end of the muscles in place, and the muscles, contracting, will draw their *lower* end upward. (Unless you genuinely want that, this reflex contraction of muscles at the back of the neck will pull the head backwards and down.)

When muscles pull their lower end upwards (headwards) they exert an upward pull on those structures immediately underneath, and so on in a chain reaction of stretch reflexes. But of course this doesn't make gravity go away – it continues to act on the other end of the structure, the feet (and buttocks, if you are sitting) just as usual. Hence the chain of stretch reflexes performs the useful function of taking up slack, bringing the muscles into a state where they are just sufficiently taut to be ready for efficient action. (**Chapter 7**)

Now look at the front of the body (figs. 33–4). Starting from the pubis, we have a pair of large muscles *(rectus abdominis)* whose fibres run vertically to attach themselves to the ribcage and to the bottom end of the breastbone. Continuing on up, we find another pair of muscles *(sternocleidomastoid)* each joined at the lower end to the top of the breastbone (and to the collar-bone). The upper end of this muscle is attached to the back of the skull, just behind the ears *(mastoid process)* and continuing backwards to lie on the occiput alongside *trapezius*. Consider the significance of the sequence *pubis, rectus abdominis, ribcage-and-breastbone, sternocleidomastoid, mastoid process-and-occiput*, which links the whole front of the torso to the part of the head that is *behind* the head-atlas joint. Via this sequence, when the head is free to balance itself, the natural rise of the back of the head can exert a lifting tendency on the front of the body, as well as on the back.

The muscles mentioned are by no means the only ones involved – just some of the most obvious. There are also interior sequences of muscles, as I mentioned before (**in Chapter 8**); they, too, are subject to this same lifting tendency, because they, too, are attached ultimately to the skull, on the inside, behind the centre of gravity.[1]

What it amounts to is the astounding fact that in what we mistakenly think of as our struggle against gravity, **our principal ally is: gravity**! For this reason, I sometimes speak

112

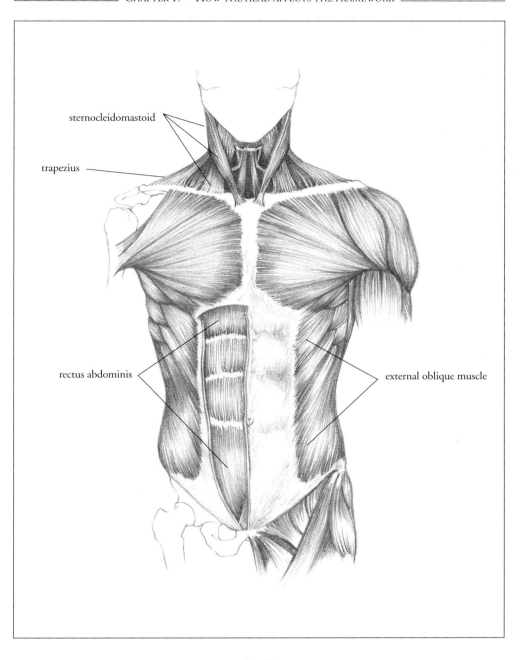

— Fig. 33 —
Front muscles

of 'letting the head fall upwards' – which is not as nonsensical as it sounds. Think of it: the effect of yielding the head to the force of gravity can be to help us up against gravity. A brilliant bit of engineering!

And that's not all. In fig. 30 we are looking at layers of back muscles that lie nearer the surface than those in figs. 31–2. Note how *trapezius* connects the *head, shoulder-blades and spinal column. Look again at the front view* (figs. 33–4): *trapezius* also makes the connection *head/collar-bone. Sternocleidomastoid* also connects *head/collar-bone*, as well as *head/breastbone.* Thus the shoulder girdle (i.e. the shoulder-blades and collar-bones) is also included in the lift made possible by the release of the head. Since the arms are suspended from the shoulder girdle, this lift will make the arms themselves seem less of a burden; the same applies to anything the hands may need to carry.

The head, you see, is part, a very significant part, of the framework. Indeed, we may say that the whole structure is in a sense suspended from the head.

Once people have understood that the head really matters in all questions of co-ordination, they often make the mistake of asking: 'Is my head in the right position now?' *This is the wrong question!* The 'right position' changes so rapidly and so subtly that only the reflexes can take care of it. I find it better to avoid the word *position*, because equilibrium is forever being disturbed, not only by obvious movements of limbs and trunk, but even by such functions as breathing and the beating of the heart. Hence, relationships between parts of the body are continually being modified. The notion of 'right positions' limits the scope and subtlety of such modifications; it is more useful to think in terms of *preferable tendencies*.

Equilibrium, according to the *Oxford English Dictionary*, is 'the condition of equal balance between opposing forces'. (It might be argued that glue is a force – but our ordinary speech respects the difference between things that are balanced, and things that are glued together!) In the human body, it is the availability of joints that allows us to pass from one balanced attitude to the next. The availability of the head-atlas joint facilitates the entire balancing process so much that no fixed head 'position' can ever be 'right'. Note, however, that this also means that you cannot be 'right' by fidgeting about trying to prove that your head is free: anxious seeking after a 'relaxed' state will preclude the spontaneous action of the reflexes. The key concept in all this is *availability for balance*.

When the head is allowed to balance as I have described, gravity, continuing to exert its pull on the rest of the body, can also provide the other end of the stretch needed by our muscles. Seeking an image, one might almost picture oneself as being slung – as if one were a sort of vertical hammock – between the effect of gravity on the head, and the effect of gravity on the feet ... but if this image doesn't say anything to you, forget it for now! It may perhaps explain itself later (when you come to try experiments 4 and 5 in Chapter 25).

If the only influence on the body were the *upward* one resulting from the effect of gravity on a freely poised head, we shouldn't be much better off. Remember that muscles, to be really efficient, must be slightly stretched. That is why, while insisting on the importance of the head, I keep saying that the head *can* have this effect. It's not a foregone conclusion. Good use of the head is primary, indispensable, because of the way

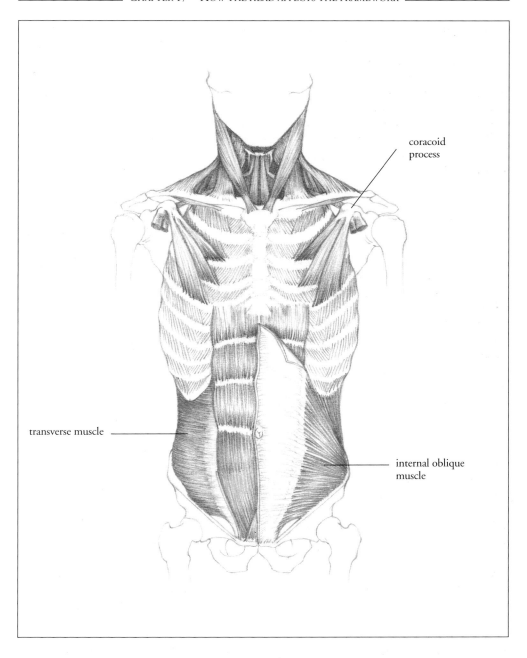

coracoid
process

transverse muscle

internal oblique
muscle

_ *Fig. 34* _
Front muscles: deep layers

115

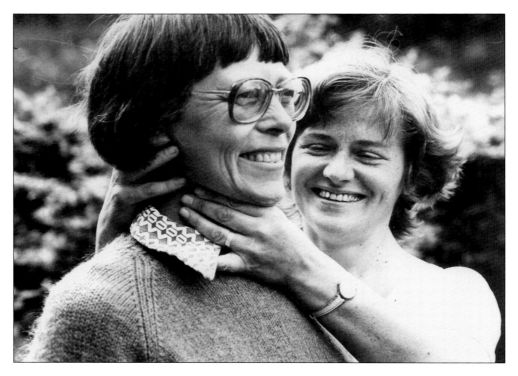

_ Fig. 35 _

Good use of the head is primary, indispensable...

it lifts and organizes our verticality. But it is not only the upward tendency that has importance. I often quote a colleague of mine who coined the saying, 'Every piece of elastic has two ends'. Contrary to popular belief, we can't really build the co-ordination we should like by starting from the ground and working up. The influence of the head is too important for that. But if *first* we pay attention to the head's freedom to balance itself, we have some choice in how we arrange things underneath it.

In discussing other matters, we shall necessarily refer frequently to the head; its inescapable influence will become clearer as we go on looking at other aspects of the structure and the way we use it. If I have convinced you of the inevitable effect of head balance on everything we do, a look at 'the other end of the elastic' awaits us in Chapter 18.

---

1. Attachments from the styloid process of the temporal bone to the hyoid bone, pharynx, and thyroid cartilage partly explain the favourable influence that habitually good head balance can exert on respiration and phonation.

THE OTHER END OF THE ELASTIC

> There had been a time when two people had thought Mr Polly the most wonderful and adorable thing in the world, had kissed his toe-nails, saying 'myum, myum!' and marvelled at the exquisite softness and delicacy of his hair ... had disputed whether the sound he had just made was just da da, or truly and intentionally dadda ... these two people had worshipped him from the crown of his head to the soles of his exquisite feet.
>
> H.G. Wells *The History of Mr Polly*

> There is enough sadness in the world without having fellows like Gussie Fink-Nottle going about in sea-boots.
>
> P.G. Wodehouse *Right Ho, Jeeves*

When we think about the 'elastic' that starts from the head, the other end is obviously – the feet. And there are several significant facts about them worth stating or re-stating. Perhaps we most often think of our feet as the things that support us. But feet are much more than supports: they are also to be thought of as *antennae* – sensory organs, feelers, if you like. Feet are receptors of a continuous flood of information about the terrain: bumpy or level, flat or sloping, gritty or slippery, solid or yielding, and so forth. It is important to us to know these things and it is through our feet that we receive an enormous amount of the moment-by-moment reporting that is needed to keep us up to date on current conditions.

If we were obliged to respond consciously to every bit of information picked up by these 'antennae', the distraction would be overwhelming. Fortunately, many of the messages are dealt with reflexly, without ever reaching consciousness – how else could we walk on uneven ground while carrying on a conversation? But all the messages must be received and understood at some level, so it is a great mistake to do anything to impede the free flow of information.

Of course our feet need protection from cold, dirt and things that might damage them. So do hands, but we recognize that the gloves which protect our hands also limit precision in our use of them, because we can't quite feel what we are doing. The German for glove is *handschuh*: 'hand-shoe'. I often wish we thought of shoes as 'foot-gloves' – then we might abandon some of the daft objects we put on our feet.

Feet, considered as antennae, are much more like hands than we realize. How can a message be expected to get through via a foot that is rendered unreceptive by clogs or platform soles? How can a foot pass on vital information if all its capability is absorbed in balancing on a high heel? How can it respond freely and efficiently if confused by discomfort? Would you mete out such treatment to those dear little feet with which you came into the world? Those same exquisite little feet, having become part of your precision equipment for balancing yourself, are even now doing their best to serve you. How can you best help them to help you?

I think you should start from a recognition that 'nature knows best'. Granted that we like to have some protection, in a good shoe we can still approximate to the bare-foot state. That is, we can feel, we can move, we can balance, we are not compelled to make unnecessary movements. The good shoe is flexible, stays on the foot and is not thicker or heavier than circumstances demand. (I am not suggesting fell-walking in ballet slippers!)

When I was young, shoes were sharply divided into 'sensible' and 'smart'. 'Sensible' shoes were heavy and clumsy looking; they seemed to have 'country walk' written all over them and no girl with any dress sense could have borne to wear them in town. 'Smart' shoes had pointed toes, which were not so bad if the shoes were expensive enough to be well made – in that case the point came beyond the actual toes.

But 'smart' shoes also had *heels*, fairly high or very high. Now, in a shoe which raises your heels above the level of your toes, a lot of your weight is thrown forward on to the balls of your feet, instead of being distributed evenly over the (already small) base of your whole foot. The resulting balance problem virtually obliges you to bend backwards at the waist. This serves the purpose of bringing your upper body backwards to compensate for the too-forward placing of legs and pelvis – but balance is maintained at the price of an exaggerated lumbar curve and gradual damage to the spinal column.

By the time a couple of generations of women had been physically distorted in this way, we were ready for the supreme stupidity of the stiletto heel. And so far out of touch with reality were we all by then that more was heard about the damage to floors and lawns than about the damage to people! Furthermore, a new generation of little girls observed unconsciously that this distortion, this deformity, was *the grown-up way to stand!*

And now, the harm is done. Postural faults of a previous generation have become installed in the body-image of today's young people. Although many of the younger generation now sensibly prefer comfortable shoes that *allow* them to move naturally, it will take more than that to ensure that they actually do so, more than that to undo the damage. (We have to admit that this deterioration was due to female folly but men, too, must accept some of the responsibility – the protruding female buttocks, the sway-back and the wobbly walk that went with the deformity, however undignified, were considered 'sexy' by some men!)

The stiletto heel makes periodic attempts at a come-back. Let's not be conned again! Resistance is easier nowadays. The young seem to feel quite well-dressed in 'trainers'; and women seeking elegance can find it, if they look around a bit, in flat or low-heeled shoes, either smart or dainty. If you do fall for a high-heeled shoe (one with a fairly robust heel, of course) ask yourself if it is really worth sacrificing the attractiveness and energy that belong to graceful, easy movement. And if (we are all human) the answer seems to be 'yes', know what you are doing and decide that these are shoes for a special occasion when you will just sit around looking decorative for a few hours. Promise yourself that you will never wear them all day, never on consecutive days – and that you will never walk further in them than from the car to your host's front door.

What if you honestly find low-heeled shoes uncomfortable, even those that look good on you? Perhaps muscles in your calves and elsewhere have already become shortened by wearing high heels for some years. In this case, you had better re-educate yourself gently. A good plan would be to start wearing *slightly* lower heels *some of the time;* next time buy some a bit lower still, and so on. You could also try sometimes giving yourself the luxury of walking around your home without shoes for short periods. For many people with this difficulty, the pleasant sensation of bare feet on carpet seems to encourage a general easing of leg muscles. If this is not your case, just be patient – the human body is very adaptable if it is not bullied!

A prevalent example of what I call bullying is to be found in so-called *exercise sandals* and other shoes similarly designed to force us to have arches where the makers think we ought to have them. Before I knew better, I once went out to buy a pair, but quickly discovered that this was just not possible – my arches didn't coincide with the lumps in the sandals. I consider that I was fortunate.

Now that I know more about it, I wonder why so many people imagine they have 'flat feet' and therefore think they need this form of 'exercise'. If your wet feet on the bathroom floor leave prints showing the little gaps that indicate the presence of arches, you have no need to worry on this score – so don't give it another thought. On the other hand, if your foot-print shows absolutely no suggestion of an arch... I am glad you are reading this book! Because you should certainly be giving some thought to your entire way of using yourself. *You can't correct feet all by themselves.* The arches in your feet are supposed to be springy, responding to what goes on above them, as well as to the feel of the ground beneath them. Not only 'flat' feet, but also very *high* arches denote a lack of springiness and are associated with problems – but this is rarely mentioned, not having found its way into folklore. I repeat: *nothing is to be gained by imposing a shape on your feet.* What is involved is your way of using the entire structure of the body – not least the head. (**See Chapter 17.**)

Another serious objection to such supposedly beneficial shoes and sandals is the *kind* of exercise they impose on the feet. With nothing around the heel to keep your shoes on, you are obliged to pick them up with each step, or else to shuffle everywhere you go. It sounds like the witch's curse in a fairy tale! Imagine a comparable 'exercise' of the hand, if something forced you to grasp every single thing you touch. What kind of exercise would it be that trained your hand to give up all subtlety of feeling, all ability to adapt to the wish to stroke a kitten, to feel the quality of silk, to pick up an egg without breaking it – abandoning all the natural possibilities in favour of an inevitable clutching reaction?

Yet at least one must admit that clutching is one normal, indeed important function of the *hand*. Can the same be said of the foot? I can pick up small objects with my feet, for fun or out of laziness, but I'd hardly say it is their main function, would you? Why should I exercise them in this way? The constant picking up of a shoe that is *made to fall off* leads to a tremendous amount of undesirable tension, impeding proper functioning of the feet and legs. Years ago, in the *Guardian*, I read an account of an article in the *Lancet*, which warned that 'more and more patients are appearing ... with pain in the feet, mostly girls in their late teens and early twenties who have been wearing the sandals...' Yet the superstition persists that something that has the word 'exercise' attached to it must be good for you.

No, the proper work of feet consists of *sensing and balancing*. The feet get good exercise by performing these natural functions in a natural way, at the bottom end of a well co-ordinated body. Away with all shoes and sandals that require the feet to do anything else! As Bertie Wooster might have said, there is enough sadness in the world without people going about in exercise sandals.

For similar reasons, it is also inadvisable to flap around in slippers that are so loose that your feet have to work to keep them on. Obviously, this applies to mules and 'flip-flops'. This type of foot-wear has a limited usefulness if kept strictly in its place – i.e. bathroom and pool-side. Even so, be careful: nasty accidents have been caused by floppy slippers as well as by exercise sandals. They can get unexpectedly caught in things or stepped on by somebody walking behind you – or even by your own other foot.

A few years ago, there was an even pottier invention than the exercise sandal. Somebody had the brilliant idea that since high heels are bad for you, heels that are too low must be extra good! So they made shoes with the toe end built up so that the heel was lower than the toe. These were known as 'earth shoes' and were a perfect example of the faulty reasoning that if something is wrong, its opposite must be right. *The argument* was that prints of bare feet in the sand often show a heavily dug-in heel; this was therefore declared to be 'natural'. *The objections* are as follows. 1) Can anyone show me that sand is more natural than rock, say, or firm soil? I repeat, our feet are designed to adapt to the conditions they find. 2) Sand is one of the more tiring surfaces to walk on. 3) People with really good co-ordination tread rather lightly – you can see that in the sand, too, if you are looking for it! So what is the point of a shoe that takes bad co-ordination for its model?

So much for that particular fad and its accompanying dangers to the Achilles tendon, the calf muscles and the general organization of balance throughout the body. It didn't catch on – but be warned! Somebody will no doubt disinter the idea next time they are trying to think up a way of getting us to spend our money. (P.S. Since I wrote this, they have! The name has changed; the objections hold.)

While we are on the subject of shoes, a word about running shoes. These are often very good for all sorts of everyday uses. But I think one had better beware of those that try to be too clever. There has been a craze for building up the back of the ankle. This is supposed to 'protect the Achilles tendon'. Perhaps some people's feet can tolerate this; often, however, the so-called protection hurts the part it is meant to help, while limiting freedom of movement at the ankle. It seems that quite a few athletes have found this troublesome, for, in an athletics magazine, I read a hint on how to deal with the problem. I pass it on here, as I found it helpful when this was the only type of running shoe I could find. You cut vertically on either side of the back seam, down to where the top of the shoe would be if it didn't have the added 'support'. The cuts are about a centimetre from the seam, so they do not make the shoe come to pieces; the unwanted piece flaps about harmlessly. I did this about ten years ago and at the same time I removed the pointless 'arch support' – an easy task, as it was only stuck in. The shoes immediately became comfortable. Though now shabby, they are still going strong on country walks. The flexible soles are thick enough to protect me from the cobbled lanes around where I live. Being rather firm, they are much less tiring than the over-springy, squidgy soles that are supposed to be so comfortable. Less dangerous, too: spongy comfort can lead to falls due to lack of information about the ground under our feet.

One more thing about what you put on your feet: very simply, don't pull socks or tights on so tightly that they cramp your toes. Toes often have a bad habit of curling themselves up – they don't need any added encouragement to do so. Of course, when I say that, I mean that the *owner* of the toes has acquired this habit. Toes can make fine adjustments to balance, so it is best not to ask them to do meaningless movements that make them unavailable for this function.

Another, very prevalent way in which people misuse their feet comes, I think, from a misunderstanding. It is commonly believed that the heel should touch the ground before the rest of the foot. The truth is that it all depends. The main factors are 1) whether you are walking up-hill, down-hill or on the flat; 2) whether you are walking quickly or slowly; 3) whether you are taking short steps or big strides; 4) how high your heels are. All of which sounds rather complicated, but isn't really, if you just decide that the feet themselves know how to be feet.

Here are some experiments, designed to give your feet the chance to forget any ill-founded instructions you may have been given as a child. Do the experiments barefoot, to begin with. Later, you should be able to incorporate the same experience in moving about with shoes on.

❏ *Experiment 1*

Sitting on a chair, toes and heels on the floor, lift one leg so that the foot slightly clears the ground. Try to make sure that the foot is just hanging freely from the ankle. Then lower the leg, allowing the floor to arrange the foot as it lands. Try not to prepare the foot in mid-air for its contact with the floor! (This is not always quite as easy as it sounds – there are so many habits involved.) Repeat with the other foot, then alternate the feet a few times.

❏ *Experiment 2*

Standing, repeat the same procedure. It may be a good idea to rest your hand lightly on a chair-back or shelf of convenient height, so as to avoid any preoccupation with balance. The feet and ankles should be as passive as possible. Looking down at your feet will interfere with the co-ordination of your upper body, so it is better to use a mirror.

❏ *Experiment 3*

Walk across the room at various speeds, *still trying not to re-arrange your foot when it is off the ground.* Many people have been so brain-washed by the 'pick up your feet, walk heel-

and-toe' nonsense that they can't manage this at once, so be patient with yourself. If you really manage to leave your feet to look after themselves, you may be able to observe some interesting things.

3(a) Walk really slowly and casually, as though you were window-shopping. It may happen that the ball of your foot touches the ground slightly before the heel does.

3(b) If you walk a little faster, with small steps, you may find that ball and heel touch down more or less simultaneously.

3(c) A bigger stride may bring your heel down first.

3(d) Repeat these three experiments with your shoes on. Unless the shoes are totally without heels, this makes a difference. Can you say what the difference is? Don't try to prove anything – just experiment and observe.

I warn you that it is not easy to be the detached observer of what you yourself are doing! For instance, if you look down at your feet to see what they are doing, you can hardly call that observing what they do naturally. I suggest you pretend to yourself that you are really strolling, hurrying, etc. and ask an objective friend to watch what really happens. Mirrors are useful, too.

I don't want to lay down rules about these things – that would be to encourage you out of the frying-pan into the fire. I just want to draw your attention to the fact that, left to their own devices, your feet are capable of greater subtlety of reaction than you may have supposed. It will be worth trying these experiments again after studying the chapters that deal with legs. (**Chapters 20–22**)

CHAPTER 19

ABOUT JOINTS
(especially those in the legs)

> To take a step is an affair, not of this or that limb solely,
> but of the total neuro-muscular activity of the moment –
> not least of the head and neck.
>
> Sir Charles Sherrington *The Endeavour of Jean Fernel*

Discussion of feet leads us inevitably to think about legs. For feet can be said to be the 'business end' of legs – or, if you prefer to look at it that way, your legs are the equipment for putting your feet where you want them. (The practical importance of the obvious is often underestimated.)

When we come to think about legs, one of the most obvious facts about them is that they are jointed. So let us think a little about what that means to us from a practical point of view. Watching herons or other long-legged birds, many of us have the impression that everything seems to bend the wrong way. Many people are also thoroughly mixed up about how their own legs work! This creates a whole lot of unnecessary difficulties.

How many times have we all heard it said that it is dangerous to lift a heavy weight with your legs straight and your back curved! I don't suppose there can be many people who are unaware of this. So why do so many people do it? They freely admit that they 'know they should bend their knees' – but somehow they forget to, or don't seem able to. They say they are 'stiff' – implying that something is wrong with the equipment. In fact, what is wrong is simply that, whereas they know that the knees should be bent, they don't really know how to bring this about comfortably.

In fact, it is not very practical to try to bend the knees without reference to all the other parts involved. So let's take a look at how the equipment is supposed to work. Shin, calf, ankle, knee, thigh, hip – how do all these bits behave when they are in movement? Perhaps we get muddled because both everyday language and (surprisingly) anatomical terminology leave a fair amount of room for confusion – so, in this chapter especially, I shall make no apology for taking extra care over defining terms.

The *Shorter Oxford English Dictionary* gives:

Joint A junction. A joining of two bones ... either rigidly or (especially) so as to move upon one another; an articulation. That wherein or whereby two members or elements of an artificial structure or

123

mechanism are joined or fitted together, either so as to be rigidly fixed (as e.g. bricks, stones, lengths of pipe etc.) or as in a hinge, pivot, swivel.

There seems to be something lacking in the language here. Personally, I feel the practical need of two different words to mean two things so essentially different. Whether we are talking about a living body or about an 'artificial structure or mechanism', it does seem strange that we cannot easily make the distinction between 'things that are *meant to move* upon one another' and 'things that are fitted together so as to be *rigidly fixed*'.

The dictionary, of course, lists all the everyday meanings. Yet even when we turn to the anatomists in search of clear expressions, we are not much better off. The detailed structure of the various joints in the human body is complex and fascinating. There are excellent books that tell us a great deal about them – more, indeed, that most of us need to know. Yet it has been pointed out (in Gray's *Anatomy*, no less) that current descriptions are unsatisfactory:

> The conventional classification ... fails to emphasize the basic mechanical difference between joints at which rigid skeletal elements are able to move relative to each other through the interposition of a deformable tissue ... and those where movement is dependent upon opposed sliding surfaces. In engineering practice this distinction is obvious.[1]

There are many complexities that the authors of Gray's would have to consider before making radical alterations in the accepted terminology; one understands their hesitation. My task is different from theirs. This is an owner's handbook, not one for technicians. Gray's and the *O.E.D.* are agreed that joints are meeting-places of bones. There are meeting-places that are not available to us for voluntary movement; these are not my main concern. My job is to try to make clear a) where the possibility of movement exists, b) the nature of that movement, and c) how it relates to movements elsewhere in the body. So when I say 'joint', unless I specifically state otherwise, I mean a place where a bone can move in relation to another bone.

We all possess certain joints that are designed to allow specific movements without compromising the healthy structure of the framework. By understanding the true possibilities of such joints, we can avoid exaggerated movement in places where all that is possible is a certain amount of 'give' in the framework. That is, we can learn to use and not misuse our joints. We can recognize *avoidable* wear and tear for what it is, and need not accept it as '*fair*' wear and tear'. Yes, here we are again, still well and truly within that eternal triangle of interdependent Structure, Functioning and Use. Those who have followed me this far will recognize that the only way we can influence what happens to our joints is via our muscles; and that how we use our muscles is fundamentally a matter of choice: a choice largely determined by our understanding (or lack of it) of the functioning of the structure as a whole.

The design of our joints is such that the bones are cushioned and protected pretty efficiently from the damage they could otherwise inflict on each other through friction and pressure. Whether these design precautions will prove adequate in individual cases will depend largely on the performance of the entire structure: on the use we make of the whole body. Joints are elaborately designed both to permit movement and to limit it. Clearly, when we talk about freedom of movement, we do not mean that bones should be able to go any-old-where, for that would mean a lack of structure, the collapse of the framework. The limitations are part of the excellence of the total design.

For instance, between adjacent vertebrae of the neck, thorax and lumbar region, a certain amount of movement is provided for, but the design of intervertebral joints puts fairly strict limits on it. Much back pain, not to mention structural damage, is caused by a lack of respect for these limits. Muscle action can modify the shape of the spinal column; but the spine is such an important part of the framework that such modifications should only be in the nature of fine tuning. Too often they become the principal means of making movements which could be achieved more efficiently – and less dangerously – if the owners were properly informed as to suitable ways of using the joints in their legs.

I have already mentioned the question of lifting heavy weights. (**I shall return to it in Chapter 26.**) But in fact it is only one of a series of related problems. Why do older people often have difficulty in getting up from a chair? Why do so many people go 'oof!' when they lower themselves on to a sofa, as though they were accomplishing some great feat? Why, in the western world at least, can so few adults go into a squat while keeping their heels on the ground – a thing every toddler can do without difficulty?

All these people are trying to use their leg muscles in contradictory ways and simultaneously. They are out of balance and tensing their legs to avoid falling. The habit of pulling the head backwards further upsets the balance. (**Chapter 17**) Whether the desired movement is with or against gravity, all possibility of a reasonable, easy use of the leg joints is thus ruled out. There is so much confusion about this that even in doctors' waiting-rooms one sees posters which, though perfectly correct as to the warnings they give, mislead by proposing alternatives that could scarcely be performed by anyone in need of the advice in the first place. Presently we shall take a good look at what is really involved in these movements of lowering or lifting oneself (with or without an external weight added to the weight of one's own body). First, a few more definitions from the *O.E.D.*

Ankle – The joint which connects the foot with the leg. (We shall ignore the secondary meaning of 'the slender part between this and the calf'.)
Calf – The fleshy hinder part of the shank of the leg.
Shank – That part of the leg which extends from the knee to the ankle; the tibia or shin-bone.
Shin – The front part of the human leg between the knee and the ankle.
Knee – The joint between the thigh and the lower leg. (The *O.E.D.* gives also 'or region about the joint' – you see how confusion confronts us everywhere! So I shall use 'knee joint' where clarity seems to require it.)
Thigh – The upper part of the leg from the hip to the knee.
Hip, hip-bone, hip-joint – Here we really start to climb the Tower of Babel, with the dictionary reflecting all the muddle that exists in people's thought and speech. (**We touched on this in Chapter 4, you may remember.**) I am not blaming the dictionary, which exists to list all the meanings given to words. From the mass of confusion and contradiction, I shall select only the definitions I am going to use.

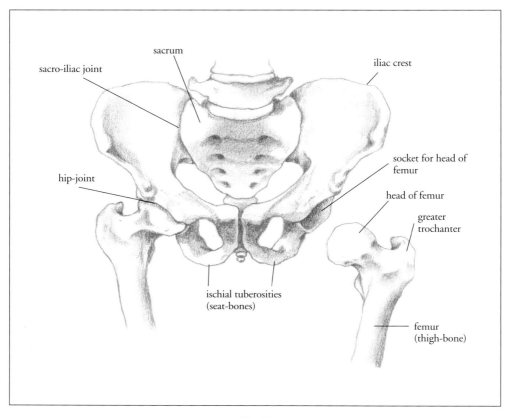

— *Fig. 36* —
Pelvis and thigh-bone

Hip-bone (also called the innominate bone) – a union of three original bones, *ilium, ischium* and *pubis*. This is a large bone of complicated shape. There are a pair of them, which meet in the middle in front *(pubic symphysis)*; at the back they articulate with the *sacrum* (i.e. the five fused vertebrae below the lumbar part of the spinal column) at the *sacro-iliac joint* (fig. 36). The sacro-iliac joint allows a certain amount of 'give' but not much movement; it can give trouble if liberties are taken with it. Hormonal changes in pregnancy render it a bit more mobile so as to accommodate the growing baby – and make it all the more important to avoid damage in this area.

The hip-bone is rather difficult to visualize, so I shall try to help you to identify bits of it in yourself. When a P.E. instructor says 'hands on hips', he means the *iliac crests*, i.e. the top of the hip-bones, nowhere near the hip-*joints* please note! **(See Chapter 4, figs. 11–12.)** When an Alexander teacher talks about the 'seat-bones', he means the bottom of the same bones, the *ischial tuberosities*. Between these upper and lower extremes, facing

126

outwards and slightly forwards is the socket for the head of the thigh-bone or *femur*. This meeting-place of the thigh-bone and the hip-bone is the **hip-joint**. It is not easy to find by touch but if you feel around while moving your leg you can probably get somewhere near by feeling which bit moves while the hip-bone stays still. The knob you feel moving is probably the *greater trochanter* (fig. 36). The head of the thigh-bone is just a bit higher and further in; you can't feel it with your fingers because it is securely held in its socket, but held in such a way that it can move about in there all right.

Hip-joints are the places where you can move your legs in relation to your body, *or your body in relation to your legs*. Mistakes, misuse here can cost us dear; there are important choices to be made and not many people are really aware of them. There can be confusion about what it is advisable to ask of this and other joints, even about what is possible. Also, it is not always obvious when and where a given movement is to be *caused* and in which joints (and in what circumstances) it is merely to be *allowed to occur*. Both actively causing and passively permitting joint function are important aspects of movement. It is good to be clear which is which. (**Chapters 20–23**) Contrary to popular belief, many of the problems people have with their joints are not due to the joints as such, so much as to muddled ideas as to how to use them. (Fig. 37)

I once witnessed a striking example of this, worth quoting here. It concerns a woman of about sixty, who had had operations to replace both hip-joints: on one side, the operation had been unsuccessful and had been repeated. This meant that the poor woman had been unable to move about for quite a long time and when she eventually tried to walk again, with joints that were now in order, she simply couldn't manage it, despite brave efforts. She came to me on crutches, the day she had been told categorically that she would never walk without them again. She kept repeating despairingly, 'I am so weak.'

With a trained assistant helping me, I managed to support her through just three steps. It was much harder work than simply carrying her would have been – so much so, indeed, that we were both drenched in sweat. 'You are not weak', I told her. 'You are a very strong woman and you are sending all your strength in exactly the wrong direction.' I remember that I shouted at her in my keenness to get through to her, to penetrate all her terrible discouragement. That was enough for that brave and determined woman. She understood and co-operated so well that on the third consecutive day of our work together, she walked upstairs at a normal pace. On the fourth day I had the delight of seeing her walk away, using her legs absolutely correctly. The street was slippery, so she was resting one hand lightly on her son's arm, for reassurance; in the other hand she was swinging the redundant crutches. Not everyone has the same ability to bounce back when things have gone that far, but I tell this story because I want it to be understood that, although it is true that misunderstanding leads to misuse leads to damage, it is unwise to assume that damage has been done, or that it is irretrievable.

Pain, weakness or feelings of 'stiffness' may be simply a protective device of nature's, a warning to think again – obviously, the sooner the better. So take heart! I expect you did everything very well when you were a baby – and that can stand you in good stead when you come to think about the way you move now. You have a lot of good experience, you see, and your body cannot truly forget it. That know-how is present in you now, even if it is a bit covered up. In the following chapters, let us see if we can remove some of the more recent layers of experience and habit that seem to make the child's know-how inaccessible to the adult.

---

1. Gray's *Anatomy*, p. 388 (Introduction to Arthrology).

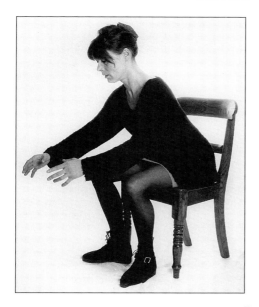

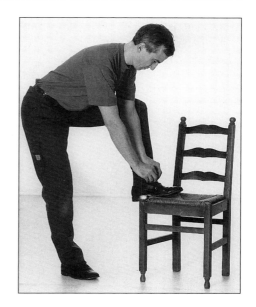

— Fig. 37a —

By understanding true possibilities of joints, we can avoid...

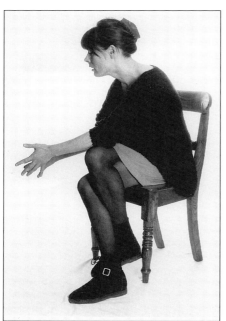

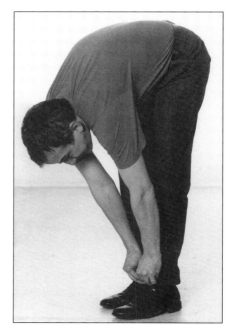

— Fig. 37b —

...exaggerated movement where there is only a bit of 'give'.

PART V
LEARNING THROUGH GUIDED EXPERIMENTATION

CHAPTER 20

LEGS: 1) LEARNING FROM BABIES

> ... at my entrance into the world... I knew by intuition those things which... I collected again by the highest reason.
>
> Thomas Traherne *Centuries*

When it comes to understanding our legs, our best teachers are very young children. So if you have a baby in the family, you are in a favoured position. If not, never mind: you have been a baby yourself, after all! So you can draw on memories and common sense in following my suggested experiments, until you have an opportunity of comparing your findings with some baby of your acquaintance.

The experiments are given in the sequence in which you probably made them the first time round. There is quite a lot to be gained from re-living them, using your adult powers of intelligent observation – and using enough imagination to put yourself in the place of a baby, without the strength, skills and experience that you now take for granted.

❏ *Experiment 1*

Lie on your back on your bed, or on the floor if you like, using a pillow under your head. (All right, babies don't need pillows, but grown-up spines are different in some ways – **see Chapter 8.**) Gently bend your knees and hip-joints, so that your thighs are more or less in contact with your abdomen. How good an imitation are you giving of a genuine baby? I bet you never saw one lying with its knees together or anything like it; the feet stay fairly close together but the little legs just flop out sideways, don't they?

If your thighs seem closer together than a baby's would be, don't on any account force them outwards: just see if you can hold on to them a bit less tightly. Gravity may change things after a moment or two. If not, never mind; your attention has been focused on the question, and that will do for now. The main purpose of this experiment is to remind you what it was like to be a baby lying on your back. Before birth, your knee joints and hip-joints had been mostly in flexion, so it was natural and easy to leave them so. Not having yet developed the muscle power that could resist the effect of gravity on your thighs, you simply let them fall outwards.

❑ *Experiment 2*

This is designed to help you think about the movements a little baby can make when lying on its front. In this position, when baby feels the need for movement, one thing he or she can do is to move the feet. When a foot is moved (there where it lies, without lifting it) whether nearer to the trunk or further away, this is achieved by modifying the angles at hip-joint and knee joint.

To try this for yourself, I suggest you push away the pillow, and lie face downwards with straight legs, feet more or less together. (Turn your head to one side if you want to.) As the leg bends, *you* may find it easy to lift your body – but you will understand that for the baby who cannot yet do this, the presence of the bed (or floor) turns the thigh outwards as the leg is folded up towards the abdomen; i.e. the head of the thigh-bone rotates in its socket at the same time as the knee joint and hip-joint are flexed. In other words, *flexion* is accompanied by *lateral rotation* of the thigh. As you experiment, leave your foot fairly central as you draw it up towards the trunk. You can then appreciate that when you straighten the leg out again, the head of the thigh-bone rotates the other way; that is to say, *extension* of hip-joint and knee joint is accompanied by *medial* rotation of the thigh.

It is important to note that the pattern of proper functioning of your hip-joints was forged once and for all by these baby movements. The basic equipment[1] was there by the time you were born; but a finishing process was taken care of by the movements you made during this early period of your life. This stage once completed, *for the rest of your life, the only way your legs can work properly, in accordance with their true nature, is when flexion is associated with lateral rotation of the head of the femur in its socket, and extension with medial rotation.* If the complications of adult life have somehow made you forget what this is like, it is well worth re-examining these movements you once did so naturally. Their availability is important to you as an adult. **(Chapters 21–23)**

❑ *Experiment 3*

See if you can make use of these same movements to shift your body along on the bed or floor. As a baby, you had plenty of motivation to make lots of these movements, for, if you flexed your legs, you could propel yourself forward by extending them, provided there was something to get a purchase on with feet or knees. Try it!

I knew a little girl at this stage of development who was lying on her tummy on the polished floor one day when she started to cry. Her mother rushed to pick her up, but I forestalled her by placing the palms of my hands gently in contact with the soles of the child's feet. Immediately, she stopped crying and started to make use of the resistance provided by my hands, to move herself across the room. The crying had apparently been born of a healthy frustration, for she plainly felt it was time to start getting about and seeing things for herself. Can you recall the feeling, or imagine it?

What with this accomplishment, plus the use of hands and arms to push your shoulder area clear of the floor, you were able to see and explore a certain amount of your environment even before you could get up on hands and knees – quite enough to make you keen to know more. Unless you were on a very slippery surface, you could make quite good progress, even with your tummy touching the ground – and you were getting stronger and more skilful all the time.

❏ *Experiment 4*

See if you can relive the great moment when you managed, with some help from your arms, to continue the movement of leg flexion/lateral rotation to the point where first one knee, then both could be brought more or less under your body. A certain amount of pressure of your palms on the floor, an effort to straighten (extend) your elbows – and you were able to enjoy a whole new perspective on the world. By this time you were well placed for making some fascinating discoveries about your body and its possibilities. The next phase suggests a further experiment.

❏ *Experiment 5*

There you were, balanced on four supports, two hands and two knees, with the backs of your feet resting on the floor behind you (fig. 38). You saw something on the ground in front of you which caught your attention – and at once your head, very heavy in comparison with the rest of you, started to pull you towards the object of interest, meeting little or no resistance from the muscles of your soft little neck. This put your balance in danger and it wasn't very nice for your wrists.

All this was a bit more than you had bargained for but luckily you discovered that your hands, not quite liking the situation and already having some experience of resisting the ground, could now try to push away this offending ground – and in so doing could push you backwards into balance again. Not only had you regained equilibrium – this was fun! But how did you manage it? I think that when you wanted your hands to resist the ground, a strong reflex reaction was stimulated in your arms, straightening them if they were slightly bent, and moving them a little backwards from the wrists. This brought about a combination of effects: the tops of your arms moved in their sockets, your trunk moved in relation to your arms, your hip-joints and knee joints became slightly more flexed.

Great! Just by giving a little pressure with your hands, you could make four pairs of joints (wrists, shoulders, hips and knees) function simultaneously. Now you could do it all over again, for there was nothing easier than to allow your heavy head to unbalance everything, and then to have the fun of putting things right again. *It was precisely because you didn't have your present muscle power that you could do all this.* Your great discovery was that you could initiate movements and then just let them happen. The hip-joints and knee joints were used passively.

We see now that 'passive' is a word applicable to other movements besides falling. Falling is passivity in relation to gravity. (**Chapter 14, experiment 2c**) *A joint can also respond passively to movement that has been actively initiated in another joint;* the response, though passive, is not necessarily gravity-assisted.

It is very important, in the interests of good co-ordination, to understand this fact. Experiment 5 presents us with a good opportunity of understanding it … so it definitely

135

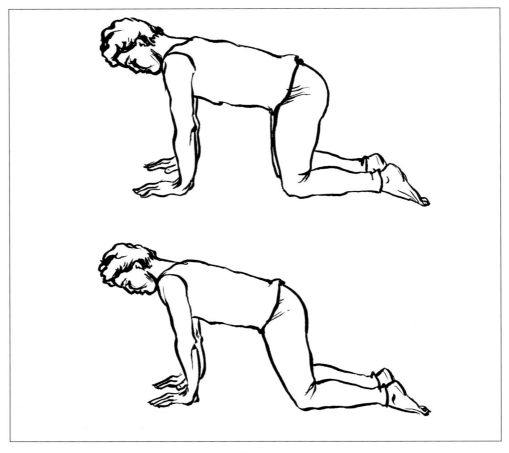

— *Fig. 38* —
Rocking on hands and knees

matters *how* you do the experiment. Don't be tempted by your adult experience into do-ing a similar movement by leg power – that is not the same thing.

When you were small, I have no doubt that you did these movements again and again, rocking backwards and forwards, looking cheerfully at everybody, inviting them to admire you and share in your pleasure. Remember? Well, perhaps not – but why not give yourself a chance to relive these moments that taught you so much about yourself?

N.B. When you make this fifth experiment, beware of letting your back sag – that is something that would never have occurred to you as a baby. Nor should you arch your back like a cat: babies have rather flat backs. Take care to start the experiment with your wrists directly under your shoulders and your knees directly under your hip-joints, your feet more or less together. The backs of the feet should rest on the floor. With vertical support from all four limbs, you now have a starting attitude from which you can very easily lose and regain balance. Remember, it was the weight of the head that started the whole rocking sequence. Don't drop the *neck*, only the head. (**See Chapter 14, experiment 4.**)

May I again remind you to avoid *deliberately* moving yourself backwards and forwards. Equally, refuse to use muscle power for the purpose of *blocking* the various joints. What we are looking for here is the easy method available to babies. The movements should happen by accident, as it were. It takes quite a lot of imagination to get the best out of these experiments. See if you can think what it must be like to have no previous experience of how all these bits of you work. Of course you *can* crawl about on all fours while making all the assumptions that your adult self is accustomed to – but then you will not discover nearly so much.

As adults we tend to forget to what extent the initiation of movement depends on interest, on curiosity, on the wish to participate in the life around us and on our sense of frustration until we can do so. These factors constitute the motive that stimulates movement. Until we understand how literally this operates in small children – how the eyes lead the head, which in turn leads the body – we shall continue to struggle to do things that were easy when we were small. The approach that was then so natural to us, if better understood, could be useful when applied to the more complex interests of our adult lives.

Grown-up people often find it hard to believe they are doing something satisfactorily unless they feel themselves making what seems to them to be a suitable amount of effort; but the accustomed feeling of 'sufficient' effort comes, all too frequently, from overcoming an habitual muscular resistance to the very thing we want to do! So another thing that can be learned from the rocking back-and-forth experiment is just how little effort is needed to move the whole body, provided contradictory efforts are not being made at the same time.

One day, while enjoying this rocking, the baby goes just too far forward, and can't push backwards. Instead, one hand is lifted and put out in front to stop the fall. At the moment the hand leaves the floor, something very important happens. To rediscover it is the purpose of our next experiment. (This one is not part of the baby's repertoire, but will help your understanding of how things work.)

❏ *Experiment 6*

Start on all fours, head not pulled backwards, wrists directly under shoulders, knees directly under hip-joints. (Don't rock for the moment; you will need time to appreciate what is happening.) Your body weight is on four points: two hands, two knees. Keeping your body still, bend your elbow so that your right hand is just lifted off the floor. Now you are on three weight-bearing points – or are you? Do it several times and notice what happens to the weight. Your left hand is bearing more weight than before, that's sure. What about your knees? What happens to them? (Please don't turn the page yet! Make the experiment yourself – my remarks can wait.)

* * * * * * * * * * * *

Most people notice increased pressure on the right knee. What about the left knee? It may take you a moment or two to realize that the pressure on that has been reduced. In fact there are now only *two* weight-bearing points, left hand and right knee. If possible, do this with a friend; a very light touch on the back (don't press!) should enable you to notice quite a lot of muscle activity there as balance adapts to the new conditions.

Can one small hand movement cause all this activity, without the owner of the muscles even being aware of it? Yes, indeed. This is one reason why it is so important for babies to crawl (to creep, in American English). The repetition of this almost imperceptible bit of exercise is a most significant preparation for the work the back will have to do when the time comes for standing upright. (It is also very beneficial for adult backs.) What is more, what we are seeing here is a prelude to walking.

❏ *Experiment 7*

When you made Experiment 6, you lifted your hand while you were stationary; however (as I mentioned at the start of this section) the baby does it while the head's weight is leading the body forwards. So the reduced pressure on the left knee has another significance. Since the hip-joints are in neutral as the body moves forward, and since the left knee is no longer pressing on the floor, a passive movement will occur in the left hip-joint, enabling the thigh to come forward into the perpendicular once more. There has been no need to lift the left knee, nor to put it down again, yet the knee has now caught up with the rest of the body. The first step has been taken! Interest in something was the motivation: the heavy head led the way; the back provided a moving bridge from which the free leg was suspended. The step itself was a passive, mechanical happening.

In the whole sequence, only the lifting of the hand was an active movement. The head continuing to lead the way, the sequence is repeated with the other hand and knee – and the forward progress continues. The forward swing of the free leg, as it moves into increased flexion, is naturally associated with lateral rotation of the head of the thigh-bone in the hip-joint, as I have explained.

N.B. To make this experiment properly, let your steps with hand and knee be small; they are incidental to the forward movement of the head. Don't lift your feet: let them trail lightly along the floor.

It is clear that there is a diagonal hand-knee support for the body throughout crawling. At first, the free hand and knee move forward separately; then, as the child gains confidence, they move simultaneously. At a later stage, bigger steps are taken, involving a combination of passive and active movements and some spiral-type trunk movements.

All this follows naturally and healthily provided there is enough opportunity for the development to occur at its own speed. For a variety of reasons, this does not always happen. Some homes don't have enough space, some floors are uncomfortable for little hands and knees, some children prefer rolling or sliding on their bottoms. And sadly, some parents are competitive about their children's progress, encouraging walking much too soon. Some of the worst backs I have seen belong to adults who did not crawl as children. *Please, never hurry a child through this stage of development.*

If the child doesn't seem interested in crawling (some aren't) invent games on the floor that involve going about on all fours. Even when walking has become the norm, don't discourage crawling if that is what the child feels like doing. And do it yourself – it is good for all sorts of things. Backs can be strengthened, period pains eased, wrists and ankles gently freed by this most natural of movements. I have even known adult cases of mild dyslexia to be resolved when the person practised crawling. I can't really explain this – it is a question for neurologists – but it seems likely that the dyslexia in these cases was an expression of slight confusion associated with the fact that the crawling stage had not been fully lived through in childhood. Here comes a useful experiment that associates hand-eye co-ordination with the hand-leg diagonals of crawling.

❏ *Experiment 8*

I hope that in your crawling experiments so far, you have been looking at the floor a little way in front of you, in order to get the 'head leading' effect. (You may have observed that babies often lift the face, but their proportions are different from ours – it wouldn't work the same for you.) For a change, try watching the moving hand as you crawl; lead with your opposite eye (**see Chapter 16, experiment 1**) and allow the head to turn to facilitate looking.

Once, at a Christmas party, I met a delightful little girl who could already walk quite well. She sat up to dinner with the adults and behaved throughout the evening like a perfect lady. About midnight, she decided to explore the apartment on all fours – and I was the person she selected to accompany her. The oldest and youngest of the company, we crawled together all over the place at a great rate. She was eighteen months old, I was sixty-five; we both enjoyed ourselves and I am sure it did us both good. Crawling is so good for one that it seems a pity to abandon it forever when one 'puts away childish things'. It is so beneficial that I think almost any crawling is better than no crawling. However, it will do you much more good if you do it thoughtfully. My remarks, all through this chapter – about imagining yourself to be a small child, finding out how your body functions without your adult experience and strength – are applicable to your crawling experiments. And the experience you gain will be helpful when we consider the movements we make as adults.

---

1. Gray's *Anatomy*, p. 350 (Osteology):
    'At birth ... the acetabulum is a cartilagenous cup...'

CHAPTER 21

LEGS: 2) LEARNING FROM TODDLERS

> Each faculty acquires fitness for its function by perform-
> ing its function; and if its function is performed for it by a
> substituted agency, none of the required adjustment of
> Nature takes place; but the Nature becomes deformed to
> fit the artificial arrangements instead of the natural ar-
> rangements.
>
> Herbert Spencer (quoted by F.M. Alexander)

When the baby, frustrated by the limitations of a view from the floor, first hauls herself to a standing position, she usually manages it by holding on to something – perhaps the bars of a play-pen, for example. In other words, she pulls from above, eyes calling on hands and arms to help the head to reach a more commanding view-point. And what helps the hands and arms to do this is: the co-ordinating weight of the head, which, as we have seen, exerts a huge influence over the rest of the body. Please note, the legs are not called upon to make what would be the immense effort of manipulating the body weight from underneath. How sensible – and how unlike adult behaviour!

So here we have our baby, clutching the rails of her play-pen. Verticality once achieved, the joints of the legs are still not braced, still not being held straight by effort on the part of leg muscles – witness the fact that the legs can fold up again without ef-fort, as soon as the baby loses her precarious balance. Here, too, there is a lesson we can learn concerning *squatting and related movements*.

We know that many adults find it difficult, even impossible, to go into the deep squat that young children find so easy and natural. Why should this be? There may be several factors, e.g. chairs. (**See Chapter 29.**) I have already hinted that misunderstandings may be responsible to a greater degree than is generally supposed and it is this aspect we shall look at now.

I am not saying that everyone should be able to do a perfect squat. If you have got through a lot of your adult life without being able to squat properly (i.e. without lifting your heels) I really don't think you should try to force yourself to do so. Quite possibly the circumstances of your life are such that you scarcely ever need or wish to perform this movement. Nevertheless, many of the movements that you do make every day could become easier as a result of understanding this baby action, so it is worth giving it some thought.

Two factors make squatting easy for toddlers. The first is the *passive use of joints*. Once a small child has achieved standing, the legs are kept straight reflexly between the weight of the body above and pressure of the floor from below – until something happens to disturb the balance. Then, security can easily be regained, nearer to the floor. Thanks to gravity and to the child's non-interference, the legs just fold passively, like a concertina, with the result that the body is lowered undisturbed.

Adults, however, often think they need to do something, to exert themselves, in order to 'stand properly'. Whatever that may mean – and there are several prevalent misinterpretations – the effort to 'stand up straight' usually results in excessive contraction of the extensor muscles controlling hip-joints and knee joints. Squatting is then thought to be a matter of 'bending the knees', and comes to involve a positive action of the muscles that *bend* the knees (knee flexors) – because far too much is being done to keep the legs *straight* (i.e. the extensor muscles are overworking). These contradictions are responsible for many of the problems that are commonly dubbed 'stiffness'.

Some people try to resolve this by standing with their knees slightly bent. But this only results in quite unnecessary contractions to stabilize the knees in their bent position! It is a fallacy to think that bent knees are more 'relaxed' than straight ones. (**See Chapter 23.**) These people, too, if they want to squat, will find themselves using muscle power to overcome their self-induced stiffness.

Toddlers, on the other hand, don't waste effort doing what gravity can do for them! The whole body is lowered safely, just because the joints of hip, knee and ankle were in an 'unprejudiced' condition and thus readily available as a set of hinges. This can work for adults, too; it all depends on balance. It may be useful to think of an anglepoise lamp, which balances in many positions without any need to tighten or loosen the hinges.

The second factor that helps young children to squat easily is *rotation of the head of the thigh-bone*. When we considered the leg movements of a baby lying down, we saw that hip-and-knee flexion is inevitably accompanied by lateral rotation of the head of the femur in its socket, and that extension is accompanied by medial rotation. The shaping of the joint has been completed by these movements and the shape does not change just because the child gets up on its feet. This is fortunate in view of the fact that very young children usually have rather protruding tummies, which would otherwise obstruct hip-joint flexion.

Of course, 'tummies' are not unknown among adults! And even the slimmest person would do well to remember that, even without this particular obstacle to hip flexion, there remains another possible hindrance: namely, the very nature of the joint itself.[1] Unfortunately, very many adults attempt hip-and-knee flexion while denying themselves the natural outward thigh rotation that should accompany it. (**See fig. 23, Chapter 13.**) This is not only unnatural in itself, but is one of the principal causes of slow, inexorable damage to the back, as you will understand as we proceed. For lack of adequate hip-joint flexion-cum-rotation, the requirements of balance oblige the spine to compensate in ways that it is not designed for.

There are cultural reasons for this widespread and dangerous mistake. Let me give you a couple of examples. During the second and third decades of the twentieth century, it became socially unacceptable for a woman to allow the natural outward thigh rotation to occur. The raising of the hemline meant that in sitting, for example, conventional decency required that the knees be held together. This was achieved by muscular contractions that ran counter to the spontaneous co-ordinating reactions prepared by nature during infancy.

It is interesting to reflect that this taboo on sitting naturally appears to have been unknown in the Victorian era (fig. 39). But in those days, a woman, seen to *cross* her legs, might well be ostracised as 'evidently no lady, my dear'! No doubt this prejudice, too, had its source in prudery, but it was certainly less damaging than the other was – *and is!* A woman could sit comfortably in her long full skirt; and if a child came crying to her, it naturally ran straight between her thighs, where she could lift it and comfort it without twisting and hurting herself as she took its weight.

Today, manners are easier – and so are styles in clothing. The mini-skirt, so limiting to freedom of movement, is still with us – but there are alternatives (fig. 40). Many woman wear trousers, of course; and at the moment of writing, longish loose skirts are again fashionable, thank goodness. Yet the habits of bad physical use remain with us, for it is easier to acquire a habit than to discard it. This may explain the widespread acceptance of jeans, which also have a restricting influence, particularly obvious in the case of the tight-fitting variety. (I have observed that even the unyielding fabric has an adverse effect on the quality of movement in many people.)

Once we had a tradition of co-ordination that was reasonable, at least in some respects. That tradition has been lost. What can be done about it? We women, whatever our age, shape or lifestyle, can take a step in the right direction (a big step for womankind!) by choosing supple fabrics and flowing styles. If designers ever happen to go back on their decision to allow comfort to be stylish, I think we should still exercise our right to please ourselves. Pretty, distinguished, or perhaps charmingly eccentric, provided we wear what suits us, we shall look nice; we'll also have a good influence on those around us – and quite possibly on fashion itself.

(It is not so difficult to influence fashion as one might think. When the platform-sole craze was at its height among the young of both sexes, I succeeded inadvertently in changing fashion throughout a sixth-form college, by dint of demonstrating to one student that she could sing better when her feet could feel the ground she was standing on. She happened to be something of a leader of fashion among her contemporaries: within weeks, plain flat sandals were all the rage, without another word from me! Surely so much demand must have influenced the local shops in their buying of stock.)

The hip-joint problem is not exclusive to women. This was a considerable puzzle to me, since (apart from the effect of jeans, common to both sexes) hip-joint misuse in men must have a different history. I discussed this with male colleagues and pupils. Remembering a time when a habit of standing with the pelvis thrust forward (virtually to the limit of hip-joint extension) seemed to be particularly typical of young American men, I sought comments on this tendency. At once I found myself in the realm of folk-lore ... One man thought the habit was due to the influence of fantasies inspired by movies about the American West. Another remembered that, during his student days in the U.S.A., it was generally held that *not* to adopt such a stance was 'an indication of sexual hang-ups'! Hang-ups or no, hyperextension of the hip-joints certainly limits freedom of movement pretty drastically. Since I first noticed it in the late sixties, the fashion has travelled eastwards and is now fairly general in Europe, affecting women as well as men.

I do not suggest that the adoption of this stance has always had similar motivation. For many people, particularly when they are tired, it simply represents a way of maintaining balance. It is true that this is one way of balancing oneself; but it is not the best way, because when the hips are in this forward position, balance requires that the ribcage be tilted backwards to compensate (fig. 41).

Hence, the lower ribs are constricted, the lumbar spine is compressed and the weight of the upper body virtually locks the hip-joints, cancelling their value as 'hinges'. Moving towards some better answers to the balance question, in the next chapter I shall suggest a few experiments, designed to help you to investigate your legs.

---

1. Gray's *Anatomy*, pp. 456–8 (Arthrology) explain the medial and lateral rotation of the femur related to arrangements existing in the knee joint.

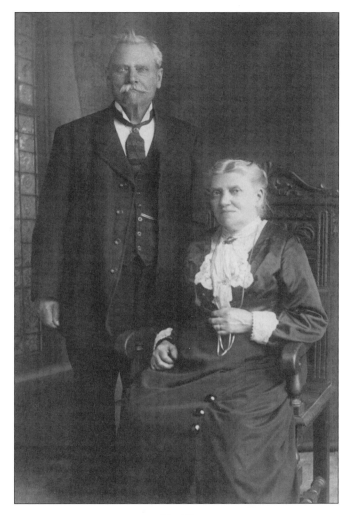

— *Fig. 39* —

In the Victorian era, convention did not require women to hold their knees together.

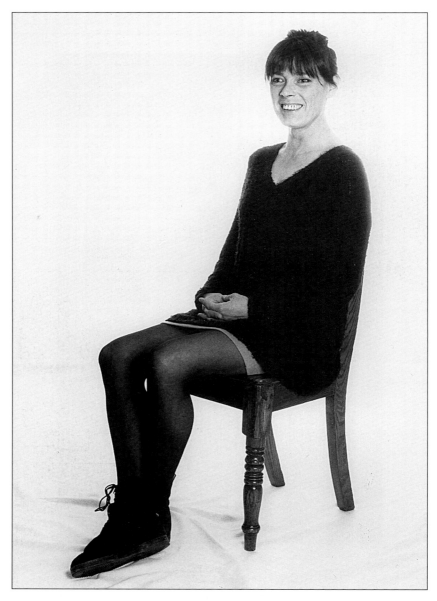

— Fig. 40a —

Mini-skirts are less easy, but with ankles crossed ... and thighs free to rotate, you may still manage to...

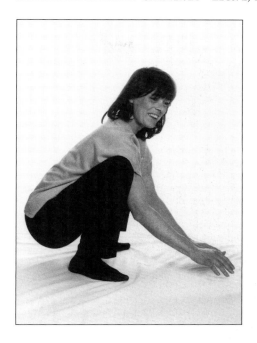

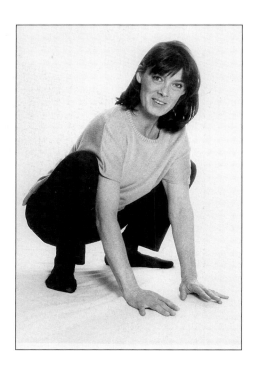

_ *Fig. 40b* _
...squat properly when you are wearing trousers again.

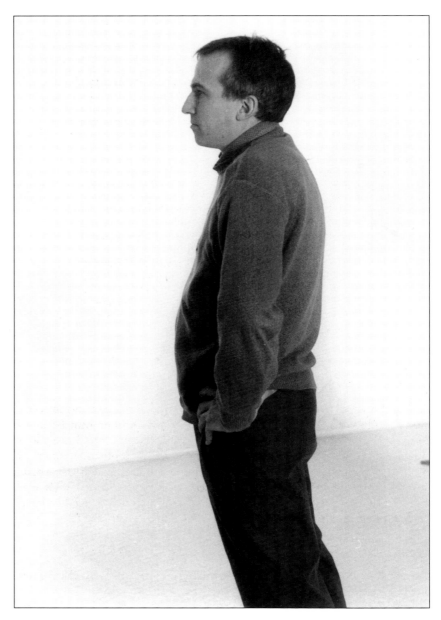

_ *Fig. 41* _
Not the best way of balancing oneself in standing

CHAPTER 22

GETTING TO KNOW ONE'S OWN LEGS

This mastery of the brain over the reflex machinery does not take the form of intermeddling with reflex details: rather it dictates to a reflex mechanism 'you may act' or 'you may not act'. The detailed execution of the motor act is still in immediate charge of the reflex.

Sir Charles Sherrington *The Endeavour of Jean Fernel*

The nibs who study these matters claim, I believe, that this has got something to do with the subconscious mind, and very possibly they may be right. I wouldn't have said off-hand that I had a subconscious mind, but I suppose I must without knowing it, and no doubt it was there, sweating away diligently at the old stand.

P.G. Wodehouse *Right Ho, Jeeves*

In exploring the leg movements we made as babies, we have already given some thought to hip-joints and knee joints. Once the baby is standing, another joint becomes important: the ankle. In good use of the legs, the three pairs of joints (hip, knee and ankle) act in co-operation. So let us now take a closer look at the possible movements our ankles offer us and then explore what is meant by this co-operation between them and the other joints. I think we can best do this by some simple experiments. (If you want to read about ankles in more anatomically detailed books, you will need to bear in mind that the lack of agreement about terminology is quite astonishing.)[1]

❏ *Experiment 1*

a) Sit in a chair and cross your left leg over the right at the knee. Bend your left ankle so that the toes come nearer to the shin. Release.
b) Place the whole foot on the floor. Leave your heel where it is and bend your ankle again – the sort of movement you might make when letting up the clutch in your car. Notice that in both cases you have made an active use of the ankle joint, so as to move the foot in relation to the lower leg.
c) Stand up and repeat movement b).

❏ *Experiment 2*

Stand facing a wall, arms at shoulder height, palms down and finger-tips touching the wall. Keeping your legs straight, and heels on the floor, allow yourself to fall forward from the ankles, until your palms are flat against the wall. Now let your elbows bend if you feel like it, but only if this is easy for the legs. Do *not* go so far that you produce a feeling of strain in the calf muscles. This is not an exercise!

Notice that the movement produced in your ankles is the same as in Experiment 1, but this time the joint was used *passively*, thanks to the effect of gravity on the rest of your body. Note also that in Experiment 1, the active use of the ankle moved the foot in relation to the leg, whereas, in Experiment 2, the *passive* use of the ankle allowed the leg, and indeed the whole body, to move in relation to the foot.

❏ *Experiment 3*

Sit down again, legs crossed at the knee. This time bend your ankle in the opposite direction – rather like a ballerina. Clearly, the movement is active and the ankle permits movement of the foot relative to the leg.

❏ *Experiment 4*

Stand in a doorway, holding on to the frame of the door to support yourself, in order to make the experiment as freely as possible without the slightest chance of falling. (You will obviously place yourself so as not to risk getting your fingers caught in the door!) Keeping the legs straight, lean backwards from the ankles, as far as is comfortable without letting your toes come off the floor.

Notice that from the ankles' point of view, so to speak, they have been through the same movement as in Experiment 3, but with a passive use of the joint. Were you surprised how much movement was possible in your ankles when you didn't have to *do* it and when there was no danger of falling? (When you might fall, instinctively you try to use your muscles to limit the movement.)

❏ *Experiment 5*

Stand in the doorway again, with your feet together. This time, stand right over to one side, so that you have room to fall sideways, using your hand or elbow to steady you and return you to the upright. How far can you go with both feet still completely on the floor?

The range of possible movement between feet and legs is quite surprising, isn't it? Paradoxically, this is perhaps why so many people fix the ankles! Freedom makes them feel as if they might fall if they allowed it to continue unchecked. So they use muscle power to limit it – and perhaps complain subsequently that they can't perform certain movements correctly because their ankles are 'too stiff'.

In one sense it may seem true that the ankles are stiff, because a habit of fixing can make muscles unable or unwilling to respond at once to suggestions that they might behave differently. But with time, patience, good use of the framework and above all, with

150

understanding of the co-ordinated action of hip, knee and ankle joints, muscles can change their little habits, like the rest of us! (Let me remind you, though, that forcing is always counter-productive. There are better solutions, as we shall see.)

Actually, 'stiffness' has very little to do with the structure of a joint (disease or accidental damage apart). *Stiffness is usually something we are doing to ourselves*, or perhaps something we have done in the past: prolonged and excessive muscle activity. It is possible to be more optimistic about it when we realize that we have some choice in the way we use our joints. This is worth emphasizing, because restricting the freedom of joints of the feet and legs is an inefficient way of trying to stop yourself from falling over!

❏ *Experiment 6*

Start by repeating Experiment 2. Do not go so far that the backs of your legs feel any strain; just notice the point at which you begin to reach the limit of what is easy and comfortable, and stop there. Now allow your knees to bend, still with weight on your hands. Take a look at your ankles. Have they bent more than was possible when your legs were straight? If not, can they do so now, if you decide to let them?

Perhaps you would agree with me that ankle behaviour depends to some extent on what the knees are doing. Let us have a look at some more experiments to do with interdependent freedom of related joints.

❏ *Experiment 7*

Stand with the feet a little way apart, keep the legs straight and bend slightly forward, from the hip-joint only. Notice what has happened to your ankles. Your legs have moved backwards from the ankles, all the way from ankle-joints to hip-joints, without you doing anything special about it. And a good thing too – it prevented you from falling, by placing your abdomen and buttocks further back, to compensate for the weight of your upper body when you moved it forward by bending. Appreciate the way your ankles and hip-joints are programmed to co-operate with each other, so as to look after your balance. And this co-operation involved the *passive* use of these two pairs of joints.

❏ *Experiment 8*

Start as for Experiment 7. After bending from the hip-joint with straight legs, see what happens if you bend your knees slightly. I think you will find it rather hard work unless you let the ankles bend a bit too, in such a way as to bring the whole structure slightly forward again. But I am sure you will find the ankles perfectly willing to co-operate with the knees, as they did with the hip-joints, in the interests of balance. It helps when you let the thigh-bones rotate outwards, in the way that we noticed when looking at baby movements. **(Chapter 20)**

❏ *Experiment 9*

Sitting on a firm chair, put your feet together and the whole under-side of the foot – toes *and* heels – on the floor. Now put your knees together; keep them there a moment, then just let the knees fall apart again. (Don't worry if there is a slight change in the foot's contact with the floor.) Do these movements a few times, always using as little muscular effort as possible.

Please notice that putting your knees together was muscular contraction. So was holding them together; both involved active use of the hip-joint. Moving your knees apart was simply a matter of ceasing to do this, i.e. of releasing the contraction: a passive use of the hip-joint. The attitude arrived at was something like a vertical equivalent of how a baby is when lying on its back.

❏ *Experiment 10*

Start as in Experiment 9, feet and knees together. See if you can move forward from the hip-joint – *without bending at the waist*. You can't go very far? That is normal. Now stop holding the knees together – and now you can continue the movement a bit further, can't you? The reason is not only that your abdomen is no longer in the way; the release makes possible the necessary lateral rotation of the head of the thigh-bone in the hip-joint. This rotation is so natural in these circumstances that it does itself, without any positive action on your part. Compare this with our experiments in baby movements. (**Chapter 20**) There is normally no real reason why it should not work just as well for adults. Trouble begins when we refuse to let it work passively.

Let me once again point out that nothing is to be gained by forcing, as if you were trying to prove something – nor by attempting to make instant improvements. Anybody can force – and live to regret it! My purpose is to help you to rediscover what you can already do very easily. Once these things become clearer to you, improvements can follow gently, at their own speed.

❏ *Experiment 11*

Start as in Experiment 10, stopping with the thighs in their fallen outwards position. Place hands on knees, to steady the knees where they are, while you lift the feet, one at a time, just enough to enable you to place them slightly apart, more or less directly under the knees. Now try moving forward from the hips, exactly as in Experiment 10. Is this easier with your feet in their new position? In any case, notice how much easier it is when you don't prevent the natural response, i.e. the rotation of the head of the thigh-bone. As you lean back towards the upright again, don't hold your thighs in their rotated-outwards position: if you leave them alone, you may find that they rotate slightly inwards.

❏ *Experiment 12*

It is also possible to move the knees further apart still, by means of a voluntary muscular contraction. In this case, there will come a point when your feet will move also, the big toe side of the foot losing contact with the floor. Play with this until you know the difference between this and the passive use of the joint. For easy movement of the legs, or of the trunk in relation to the legs, the availability of passive rotation of the hip-joint is an absolute must. Nobody can ignore this requirement without running grave risks.

In this chapter, we have been exploring the possibilities offered by the joints in our legs. In Chapter 23, we shall take a closer look at some of the ways we most often need to make use of these possibilities.

---

1. The following examples are taken from:
    I.A. Kapandji, *The Physiology of the Joints, Vol. 2, Lower Limb*, Edinburgh, Churchill Livingstone, 1974;
    F.P. Kendall and E.K. McCreary, *Muscles – Testing and Function*, Baltimore, Williams and Wilkins, 3rd edition, 1983;
    Gray's *Anatomy*;
    W. Platzer, *Color Atlas and Textbook of Human Anatomy, Vol.1, Locomotor System*, New York, Thieme, 4th English edition, 1992.
    a) What Kapandji (p. 140) calls flexion of the ankle-joint, Kendall (p. 26) says is extension. Kendall, however, like Gray's (p. 461) prefers the term dorsiflexion.
    b) What Kapandji calls extension of the ankle-joint, Kendall says is flexion; plantar flexion being the term employed, however, in both Gray's and Kendall. Kapandji maintains that plantar flexion is 'an incorrect term'.
    c) 'The ankle or the tibiotarsal joint...' (Kapandji, p. 136))
        '... the upper ankle joint or talocrural joint...' (Platzer, p. 218).
    d) '... the lower ankle joint or subtalar and talocalcaneonavicular joints...' (Platzer, p. 218)
        'Subtalar (Talocalcanean) Joint' (Kapandji, p. 158) (Note that Kapandji discusses this joint with the foot, not with the ankle.);
    Gray's (p. 463) explains: '... two articulations ... form a single functional unit which is often termed the "subtalar joint", but this term is used here for the posterior joint only, the anterior being described as part of the talocalcaneonavicular joint.'

CHAPTER 23

THE RIGHT WAY TO 'USE YOUR LEGS TO SAVE YOUR BACK'

> While reason is not divorced from the practical aims of
> life... it is not a mere tool for immediate action. Its func-
> tion is to know, to understand ... and to relate oneself to
> things by comprehending ... their hidden relationships...
>
> Erich Fromm *Man for Himself*

> As far as one can tell, then, many structural specifics are
> determined by genes, but another large number can be
> determined only by the activity of the living organism it-
> self, as it develops and continuously changes throughout
> its lifespan.
>
> Antonio Damasio *Descartes' Error*

People are often advised, especially if they suffer from back pain, to use the legs to save the back. Too often, this is understood as making the legs work harder. But unless the legs work in the right way, working them harder does them harm. Worse still, inefficient use of the legs is also detrimental to the back itself. In many cases, the legs become disproportionately strong in relation to the back; by hurrying into action, whatever the task, they often deprive the back of a bit of healthy activity that it would quite like to perform. It is a great pity to forget that every part of us can benefit from being asked to act according to its true nature and capabilities, as part of a co-ordinated team.

In this chapter, we are going to think about some ways in which we can make practical use of facts I have already explained. (**Chapters 19–22 and 13–14**) Let me begin by reminding you of what you discovered when, as a baby, you first got yourself up off the floor: that the natural way of organizing movement is to want to get the head somewhere, so as to have a better view. Every creature, since the world began, has been able, as a matter of course, to manoeuvre its head to where it could best eat, see, listen, sniff the wind for danger. All these functions belong to the head and are vital for survival, so of course it has to be a simple matter for any creature to put its head where it wants its head to be. And why should it not be equally simple for you? After all, you have millions of years of evolutionary experience behind you! When you want to put your head somewhere, you have a right to assume that the rest of your body will co-operate.

The difficulty for many of us humans is that we tend to ask ourselves how to do things – and to come up with the wrong answer, very often because we have left out of our calculations the practical, physical influence of the head on the rest of the body. Wrong answers create wrong habits create problems. I have often found that some wrong answers can be tidied away by explanation; that thoughtful experimentation can loosen the grip of habit; and that many problems can thus be shown to be less concrete than we suppose.

I should like to ask you to take another look at Chapter 14 (especially Experiment 5 and accompanying explanation) as it has an important bearing on most of my suggestions in this chapter. An understanding of the role of the head, combined with an appreciation of how the leg joints can function harmoniously, should help you to get smooth co-operation from your body whenever you want to get your head somewhere.

❏ *Experiment 1*

Sit on a firm chair, with the feet slightly apart. Where does your weight press most noticeably on the chair? Ideally, your weight should be nicely balanced on the seat-bones, the *ischial tuberosities*. (**Chapter 19**) People who make efforts to 'sit up straight' usually tilt the pelvis, exaggerating the lumbar curve ('hollowing the back', as it is often called). This places the weight of the trunk too far forward, on to the thighs, which is bad for the circulation as well as for the back. The true happy medium is not to be found by sitting like that, any more than by slumping and thus distorting your spine and abdomen and restricting your breathing. The seat-bones are well designed for sitting on in a balanced way, as they are rather like rockers; and naturally, leg movements are much less restricted when your weight is not on the thighs. When the legs are available for movement and the head is freely balanced on *its* little rockers, not pulled backwards (**Chapter** 14) this is an easy and comfortable way to remain seated.

Experience shows that a comfortable sitting position is most easily reached when the standing that precedes it is also balanced and economical. There are a few points worth mentioning about that, and here are some experiments to illustrate them. Make the experiments standing; hold on to something if you like, for balance, while you consider what is happening; use a mirror if you like, but *avoid bending to look directly at your feet or legs*.

❏ *Experiment 2*

Standing, bend one knee, so as to lift the foot behind you. Of course this demands active flexion of the knee joint. Replace the foot on the ground.

❏ *Experiment 3*

Lift one foot in front of you, as though you were about to climb a step. The hip-joint bends so that the thigh is roughly horizontal; the lower leg and foot are just dangling. This is active flexion of the hip-joint. The knee joint also is flexed, but *passively* – you didn't do it, gravity did. Now:

❏ *Experiment 4*

Still standing, let the foot fall to the ground again. Because you stopped holding the hip-joint in flexion, you now have passive extension of hip-joint and knee joint, thanks to gravity. Your weight is still on one foot; continue to think of the other leg and foot as dangling, as you sway gently to even up the weight on your feet. The 'dangling' leg coped all right, didn't it? You didn't have to do anything about it. (In fact there was a small adjustment, a tiny extra bit of extension to meet the extra weight – but it *just happened*, didn't it? There is a reflex that looks after that.)

Perhaps you are now wondering why people so often make work for themselves by *holding* hip-joints and knee joints in extension when they are standing? Do you have a habit of making unnecessary work of this? It seems a funny thing to bother to do when gravity and your reflexes can do the work for you! Let me emphasize that *in normal standing the knees should not be flexed*. That leads to stiffening in the flexed position, which is no better than stiffening in the extended position.

❏ *Experiment 5*

To make certain this last point is clear, brace your knees as much as you can, so that the kneecaps rise. Now gently allow the kneecaps to drop again, but don't bend the joints. This ensures quite enough firmness in the legs for secure standing, although you may be surprised how little effort is involved. It also provides a neutral starting-point, from which all three pairs of joints (hip, knee and ankle) can be flexed passively or actively, as appropriate.

Now I should like you to rediscover what it is like to permit yourself the passive type of flexion in all three pairs of joints simultaneously. You have made experiments to show the difference between active and passive use of the joints. You have seen that movements against gravity involve some muscular effort somewhere. You know, too, that movements assisted by gravity can look after themselves – or can they? If there is no danger of falling, they can. But if you feel yourself falling, you will obviously do something about it. The all-important question is, what? The reason many people cannot squat is the same reason that they make an inefficient – and not very graceful – fuss about lowering themselves on to a chair: they start by putting themselves in danger of falling, then fix their joints to stop themselves falling, then are unable to believe that these same joints could, if decently treated, behave as beautifully made, well-oiled hinges.[1]

We all know that something that is out of balance will fall unless something is done about it. So why do we try to sit down by putting ourselves out of balance? When you are standing in front of a chair, with the intention of sitting on it, it is obvious that your intention includes putting a lot of your weight behind your feet, i.e. outside your base. Therefore, common sense says that you will need to put quite a lot of your weight in front of your feet, i.e. outside your base in the opposite direction. To do this satisfactorily requires the co-operation of *all three pairs of joints: hip, knee, and ankle*. Fortunately, they know very well how to work as a team. Indeed, one might say they are programmed to do so. **(Remind yourself how they kept your balance for you in Experiments 7 and 8 of Chapter 22.)**

157

You may not find it easy at first to give the joints permission to do their job. If they are not used to doing things their own way, they may be hesitant. If you are not convinced they are competent, you may be sending them the sort of message that really means 'I want to let you do this movement, but for heaven's sake don't let me fall!'

This is why I should like you to be considerate to yourself when doing the next experiment. So stand with your back to a sofa, as if intending to sit – you will soon see why.

❏ *Experiment 6*

With your back to the sofa, first repeat Experiments 7 and 8 of Chapter 22. Then see if you can use the same approach to allow the joints at hip, knee and ankle to bend some more, keeping the trunk long, with no folding at the waist. If this seems difficult, perhaps you forgot that physiologically, *co-ordinated flexion of the leg joints is necessarily accompanied by hip-joint rotation* – in other words, the knees must be allowed to part as they move forward. Don't put off thinking of this until you are already bending the knees: before you start moving, give permission for the two things to happen simultaneously from the beginning of the movement. Your legs know how to do it and will thank you for not interfering.

Remember not to pull the head backwards, or your balance will suffer and your legs will start working too hard. (If you do lose balance, you know you will land on the sofa, with no harm done, so you can feel free to experiment.)

It is best not to be too ambitious, but, after you have played with this for a while, you may find you can continue using passive flexion of hip, knee and ankle joints, *still with no bending at the waist,* maintaining an easy balance until your bottom meets the sofa – it's easier if your bottom isn't feeling for the sofa before it meets it.

If this is no problem, you could try repeating the whole experiment away from the sofa – perhaps you are one of the fortunate ones and can squat like a baby. Don't try too hard, and *above all, keep your heels on the floor!* This is important: letting them come up may *seem* easier, but it puts a lot more strain on the legs and back. It is better to keep your heels down and let the joints do as much passive folding as they can do easily. Lifting your heels invalidates the experiment, creating the very imbalance and needless tension we are trying to avoid. Don't be too keen on succeeding at getting all the way down; it's more important to keep your body long and not to collapse at the waist.

If you do find yourself squatting, you will need to come up again. Try the toddlers' way (they are the experts): head down, bottom up, to give an easy start to the straightening of the legs. If this seems awkward for you, invent a way you find easier, via sitting or kneeling.

Whether squatting or coming up again, please don't force! Forcing leads to problems. Ease leads to greater ease another day. Experience shows that there is nothing to be gained by getting competitive with oneself about this kind of thing. Thirty-three years ago I couldn't squat at all. It took me six months (and help from Alexander teachers) until I could let my joints behave like proper hinges – and I have been able to squat easily ever since. Some people take longer; some can do it at once; some never get all the way –

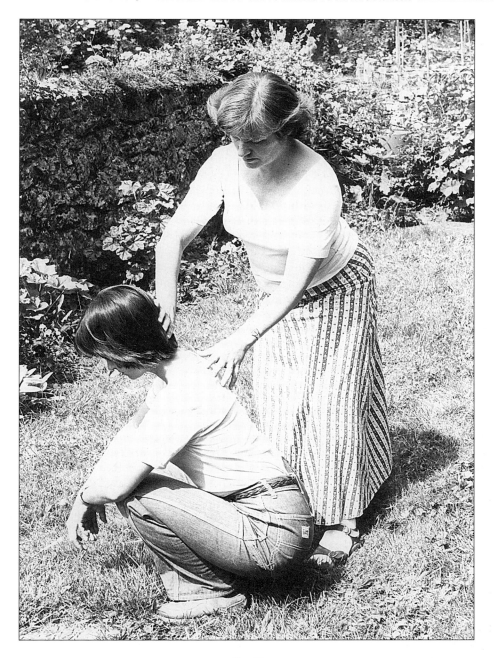

— Fig. 42 —
A perfect squat, with heels on the ground

it doesn't matter too much. What we are aiming at is not squatting as such, but an improved understanding of the movements we need in daily life.

❏ *Experiment 7*

Whatever results you had with Experiment 6, try exactly the same approach, but standing in front of an ordinary dining-room chair, with your back to it, as though you were about to sit down. Instead of sitting down, pretend you are going to squat with heels on the ground, always remembering to keep your body long without bending at the waist. Don't pull your head backwards, but let it lead you as far forward from the hip-joint as may be necessary to feel absolutely confident that you wouldn't fall, even if the chair were not there. When your passive movement reaches the point where your bottom touches the chair seat, you are sitting! All that remains is to open your hip-joint (by moving your torso backwards from the hip-joint so that you are sitting vertically).

There are considerable advantages to this way of lowering yourself on to a chair: a) perfect balance throughout the movement; b) no strain for legs or back; c) no danger of an undignified landing if the chair happens to be lower than you expected; d) a position, once you are seated, that is more comfortable, healthier for your back, digestion and breathing; e) standing up again is easier. Who would forego all these advantages in exchange for effortful verticality with the knees pressed together, followed by a tired and ungraceful slump?

❏ *Experiment 8*

Sitting in nice balance, hands by your sides, remind yourself how natural it is, in moving, to let the head of the thigh-bone rotate in its socket. Now we are going to see whether, with the help of the head, you can use even less effort than before, in making use of the hinge that the hip-joint offers. Try this time to make the moving forward process even more passive, as follows.

You are sitting with your head freely poised, of course! Before even thinking about moving from the hip-joints, release the head a little bit more forward from its joint than your sitting balance requires. NB – only the face should drop, not the neck. (**Chapter 14**)

If you are allowing your hip-joints to be really and truly available, this slight displacement of the weight of the head can have the effect of unbalancing the whole torso, so that, without any muscular effort around the hip-joint, the body will start gently tipping forward from the hip-joint – just leave it to gravity. Back muscles will automatically come into play to stop you falling further than you decide to – and this little bit of exercise is just what they like.

Don't let the mention of gravity cause you to exaggerate and make yourself heavier than you really are; gravity can cause falling without any help from you! If your head leads the way as I have described, it will prevent your body from collapsing and so from impeding the freedom of your hip-joints by putting extra pressure on them.

The movement we have just explored is useful when you are seated and want to take hold of something just out of reach on the table in front of you. It is also a preparation for an easy method of...

Standing up

Notice that what we have investigated in Experiment 8 is also a necessary component in getting up from a chair efficiently and without fuss. Let me again remind you that it is very easy when you don't prevent the natural rotation of the thigh-bones. If you have not used muscular contraction to *flex* your hip-joint, then *extending* it (as you straighten into the standing position) will be that much less work.

Let us think about that. What actually happens when you stand up? Most people seem to assume that the action must come from their feet and legs. Examine this assumption for a moment. Suppose you are confronted with a life-size doll, with the same joints as a human being. Suppose the doll is seated and your task is to get it to its feet. Do you really get down on the floor and try to manipulate the doll's legs so that they will straighten while supporting the doll's weight, most of which, don't forget, is at present behind the legs and well behind the feet? Surely not.

Such a method would never occur to you. You would grasp the doll by the upper part of its body, or by the head. Similarly, if you wanted to get a real person to stand up from a chair, you might try pulling her up by the hands or arms, or by placing your hands in her armpits and then lifting; or perhaps you would try a sudden push upwards from behind; or possibly you could ask her to lean on you in some way while you yourself stood up; in desperation you might even pull her up by the hair as in a cave-man cartoon! I can imagine all sorts of methods you might dream up. The one thing I am sure you would not attempt would be to start the whole process from her legs. Isn't there a discrepancy here between common sense and what we often do when we stand *ourselves* up?

Of course, you might have better luck if you could first get the person's weight off the chair and over the feet. Then you could try lifting – but this would not work if the legs were already stiffened in a bent position, which they would be if there were any fear of falling. And the legs would have an absurd amount of work to do if they were asked to straighten, not only under the weight of the body, but against the opposing action of their own flexor muscles. Besides that, a considerable balance problem would have been created, whose solution would probably demand quite unpleasant things of the back. These are some of the posers people set themselves every time they stand up. Are you in the habit of making the same assumptions?

A different approach is to consider where, in space, your head would be if you were already standing, and to compare this with its present whereabouts. The distance between the two placings is not so great. What about the direction? Suppose we just think about that, ignoring for now any question of how you might get up there. Standing, your head will be higher than now as you are sitting. It will also be further forward. Logically, therefore, it will be best to avoid all those movements of the head that would take it backward-and-down, or sideways-and-down, or forward-and-down. When you start by *choosing not to go in those directions*, the head is already about as near to its destination as it can be while you remain seated. Decide that it isn't worth stiffening your legs – that only puts the brake on, so to speak. Decide that the nature of the movement shall be the gentle tipping forward described in Experiment 8; as the tipping starts, steer your head towards its goal. After all, you could use the same tipping movement with the aim of looking under your chair – so why not take advantage of it to stand up and walk across the room, or to stand up while turning sideways as if to greet someone?

As I have already pointed out, it is reasonable to expect your body to co-operate in putting your head where you want it. What is unreasonable is to put difficulties in its way, which is what we do if we stiffen the legs in expectation of hard work. If the legs are available for movement, they will straighten quite easily as your head leads your body obliquely forward-and-up. When the head arrives over the feet and the legs are straight, *you are standing* – there is no need to do that little bit extra that locks the hip-joint into hyperextension. (**See Chapter 21.**)

Note that I am not saying the legs do *nothing* – but that problems come from exaggerating what they may have to do. To stand up involves moments of hip flexion and of hip-and-knee extension; if the flexion is made by muscle power it will have to be corrected by excessive muscle power – with the risk of damage in the long run. It is useful to take advantage of the possibilities implied in passive use of joints; then the active use may very well seem like nothing, or nearly nothing.

Further uses of Experiment 8

The standing position is vertical; so, usually, is good sitting. Between these two, as the legs fold on their three sets of hinges at hip, knee and ankle, the body ought not to collapse at the waist, but should slope at various angles as balance demands. Our hinged legs thus offer a multitude of monkey-like possibilities, all the way from stand to squat: these are useful in all sorts of activities, housework, gardening, doing up shoes, picking things up off the floor, washing hands at a low sink, using a low workbench, doing up a child's buttons, the list is endless. Once the principle is grasped, it can be applied endlessly to accomplish, without damage to our backs, very many of the movements most frequently needed in daily living.

Lifting things

It is particularly important to remember all this whenever there is something heavy to be lifted. Essential safety rules for lifting heavy objects are given in Chapter 26, and should be read in conjunction with this chapter.

To use your hinge-like possibilities to the full, you will of course need to start with the feet somewhat apart (how much depends on the circumstances). But don't let this fact lead you into a habit of standing or sitting with feet *exaggeratedly* wide apart, a situation in which the hip-joints could be subject to undesirable mechanical forces. The very wide stance is brought about by *abduction*, which is a different movement from the rotation I have emphasized. Here is an experiment to help you recognize the difference.

162

❏ *Experiment 9*

a) Standing with feet together, keep the heels close while you turn one foot out like a ballet dancer. Again, don't strain, but notice that the whole leg moves from the hip-joint. This is *rotation – active, in this case*. As we have seen, a small amount of *passive rotation*, in which the feet can stay put, is an essential component of good co-ordination.

b) Starting with feet together, lift one straight leg sideways, as far as you comfortably can – don't strain. This is *abduction*. I have suggested trying it like this so as to notice clearly the difference between the two movements, but of course you also use abduction when placing the feet apart – and sometimes you will combine the two.

Reading and thinking about these principles and their practical application can protect you from harmful misconceptions, thus paving the way for ease and comfort. It will be obvious from my previous remarks that a good Alexander teacher could help you to experience the confidence that comes with fluency of performance.

A word of warning

It is sometimes suggested that there is something to be gained by sliding the back up and down a wall; this is supposed in some way to free the legs, though how it could do so is not explained. I most strongly advise you *not* to try this exercise. The correct and easy use of legs is only possible where there is good balance of the whole structure of the human body, as I have explained. Sliding up and down a wall relies on the wall for support; no balance is involved and there is a risk of undesirable development of leg muscles, whose disproportionate 'strength' will most probably weaken your back. You might also hurt your knees. It has been claimed that the procedure is beneficial for the back, but this has been convincingly refuted by Walter Carrington.[2]

---

1. Between the joints of hip, knee, and foot, there are quite delicate reciprocal movements. I have not attempted to describe them, because they occur by themselves, giving no trouble when balance is properly maintained. It must be said, however, that knees undergo a good deal of pressure, and are more easily damaged than repaired. Their best protection is to work as part of a balanced team of joints, as I have indicated.

2. W. Carrington and S. Carey, *Explaining the Alexander Technique*, London, Sheildrake, 1992, pp. 89–90: '... I can't imagine why anyone thought this procedure was useful – it goes against everything that is known about basic mechanics ... the curves of the spine are vital and necessary in the whole arrangement of support, shock absorption and weight-bearing ... Flattening the spine against a wall in the upright amounts to a distortion...'

CHAPTER 24

THE SHOULDER GIRDLE

My yoke is easy and my burden is light.
Gospel according to Matthew

In Chapter 20, when we were dealing with crawling movements, we saw all four limbs as sharing the work of support and locomotion. As we grow and develop, we find that, thanks to our verticality, the complicated jointed tools consisting of hand/forearm/upper arm are thus freed for a multitude of other activities, and the work required of them becomes increasingly differentiated from the work that must be done by the foot/lower leg/upper leg piece of equipment.

In Chapter 23, we looked in some detail at the interplay between the lower limbs and the trunk, particularly with a view to taking better care of the back. Now it is time to reflect on the rather different relationships existing between the *upper* limbs and the trunk, and to see what *they* can mean to us in the practicalities of daily life.

The shoulder girdle is the yoke-like structure from which, at the shoulder-joint, the arms are suspended. When used properly, the 'yoke' is easy and the burden light. (**See Chapter 17.**) Besides being there for the arms to hang from, the shoulder girdle forms an important part of the framework of the trunk. It is superbly designed to fill this double role; nevertheless, the complexity of the arrangements can and does give rise to misunderstandings – and hence to inappropriate and damaging ways of using the equipment.

The shoulder girdle (fig. 43) consists of the two shoulder-blades and the two collarbones. Near the outermost point of each shoulder, the shoulder-blade *(scapula)* is joined to the collar-bone in such a way that movement can occur between the two bones. The collar-bones, by maintaining the distance between the shoulder joints, help to provide our arms with a wide range of movement. The only place where this combination of shoulderblades and collar-bones directly meets the skeleton of the trunk is at the *sternoclavicular joint,* i.e. where the collar-bone *(clavicle)* moves on the breastbone *(sternum).* 'The scapula floats in a muscular suspension, lightly strutted by a slender mobile clavicle.'[1]

Contrast this with the much greater solidity of the pelvic girdle, whose large hipbones meet the sacrum in a joint permitting very little movement indeed. (**Chapter 19**)

165

Whereas the pelvic girdle is massively constructed for *resistance to stress*, in the shoulder girdle both the nature of the joint and the lightness of the bones favour *mobility*.[2] This allows a vast range to our hands – our grasping, enquiring, sensitive, adaptable hands.

There are seventeen muscles attached to each shoulder-blade, connecting it directly to the head, the upper arm, the forearm, the ribcage, the spine (neck, thorax and lumbar parts) as well as to the hyoid bone (to which the root of the tongue is attached). Thus its behaviour influences and is influenced by the behaviour of all these parts. The collar-bones are connected muscularly to the head, ribs, breastbone and arms. In addition to all this, both shoulder-blades and collar-bones have surprisingly close relations with abdominal muscles.[3] Where so many muscles are involved, the combinations and permutations of their behaviour are extremely complex and allow for an enormous variety of uses – and misuses. Gray's says:

> Attention should be drawn to the fact that muscles which are antagonists for one type of movement may nevertheless combine together and act as prime movers for another. Movements and not individual muscles are represented in the cerebral motor centres, and, more significantly, muscles are not associated, in their nervous control, in unalterable partnerships, but can be combined with great plasticity as the demands of movement dictate.[4]

Small wonder that the shoulder girdle is often seen to adopt some strange attitudes! In this sea of complexity, two requirements stand out like huge rocks:

1) *The shoulder girdle is there to have arms suspended from it.* The arms are for getting our hands where we want them, which is usually somewhere where we can see what we are doing with them. The versatility of the upper limb, combined with the way our eyes are placed in the head, and with the way the head itself is articulated, ensures a wide field in which hands and eyes can co-operate. In keeping with this advantage is the fact that the *shoulder-blades, lying against the ribcage, curve slightly* forwards. Certainly this is how things are supposed to be – but unfortunately much postural advice ignores the facts.

2) *The other inescapable requirement, if the framework is to be maintained adequately, is that the shoulder girdle must remain wide enough to do what is needed for the other structures that depend on it.* This necessity may be what lies behind all those exhortations to pull our shoulders back. Doing that, however, is worse than useless: no muscle can actively widen the shoulder girdle, for no muscle can push, as you know (**Chapter 6**) and clearly there is no point from which the shoulders could be pulled out sideways. Moreover, *any attempt at improvement must respect the curved shape of the structure.* If a person is really too narrow in front, the only difference that can be achieved by pulling the shoulders back is... to make matters worse by making the back narrow, too. One must be particularly careful not to give children the wrong idea about this.

Of course, we all like to see the perfect little back and shoulders of the healthy toddler, and we can sympathize with the reaction of parents who see their school-aged child sitting slumped in front of the television. What has become of all that perfection they used to find so touching? But look what happens if they say 'You are getting round-shouldered – for goodness' sake sit up and put your shoulders back!' Young Johnny, who wants to amuse himself in peace, may appear to take heed, if only temporarily, but does not ask himself how to release the damaging muscular pulls he has been inflicting on himself: he only opposes those pulls with others, still more damaging. Already seen to be narrow in front, he now becomes narrower still, because the shoulder-blades are pulled towards each other in the back, sticking out like wings. Important muscles become too slack to do their job. The all-important muscular arrangements between shoulder, neck, head and spine have been upset and the co-ordination of the whole system crucially disturbed. On top of all that, Johnny may be left with the idea that this uncomfortable distortion of nature is what is meant by 'good posture'. (He may believe this even while returning to his slump!) No, two wrongs don't make a right, and *this approach must be discarded, for pulling the shoulders back can do serious damage* – not least by interfering with good breathing. (**Chapter 11**)

However, we cannot ignore the need for width through the whole structure, nor the fact that this need sometimes presents difficulties. If shoulders are a real problem, there is no quick remedy. But there is a solution, just one, and this is it: *the only way to restore width is, quite simply, to stop pulling the shoulders towards each other, no matter whether the narrowing appears to be in front or behind.*

Once you give up the misuse, the body's natural tendencies can start to reassert themselves. I cannot promise instant results, but as I have already pointed out, muscles are obedient things. If you decide you would really like the tips of your shoulders to go further apart, if you keep on remembering that that is what you want, and if at the same time you remember that there is no way of bringing this about by muscular doing... then, gradually, any muscles that may be holding your shoulders too close together will get the message that you want them to stop it. It is unnecessary to go into questions about exactly which muscles will be influenced by your wish to be wide. We don't have that sort of control over them. As Gray's explains in the passage quoted above, the brain centres controlling these matters are designed to deal with movements, not with individual muscles. It is important to understand that *this is a case where not doing the wrong thing is all that is required for good movement to become possible.* Once this is clear, there are ways of helping the improvement along, as we shall see. (**See also Chapters 25 and 26.**)

We tend to think of our shoulder-blades as being at the back, so it can be helpful to note that part of the shoulder-blade (the *coracoid process*) pokes forward under the collar-bone to form part of the framework of the *front* of the body (figs. 43, 34). This helps one to realize that width can only mean total width: there is no such thing as widening the front at the expense of the back or vice versa. We should also understand that widening at the back concerns muscles whose fibres run obliquely (fig. 30).[5] This means that if the curves of the spine are exaggerated there cannot be true widening – nor can there be if we slump. Either mistake would deprive some of those oblique fibres of their elasticity, by overstretching them or by imposing slackness on them. Any attempt to force the shoulders downwards is also a mistake, for the same reason – look at the direction of the muscle fibres and you will see for yourself what I mean. While you are thinking about the shoulder girdle, examine your collar-bones, or those of a friend, and notice that from the joint with the breastbone they lead, not only sideways but up and back to where they meet the shoulder-blades. (Don't be misled, by some anatomical diagrams you may come across, into thinking of the clavicles as horizontal – a diagram is not necessarily lifelike and may be illustrating some other point.)

I am not suggesting you need to do anything about all this – but a good general idea of how things are supposed to work will certainly help you to avoid mistakes. Above all, bear in mind that, since the shoulder girdle is suspended from the head (**Chapter 17**) *the whole intricate structure depends for efficient support on good head balance.* If the head is pulled backwards, an uneconomical amount of work has to be done to combat the tendency of the whole body to become collapsed and disorganized. And some of that work will almost certainly be done – quite inappropriately – by the shoulders.

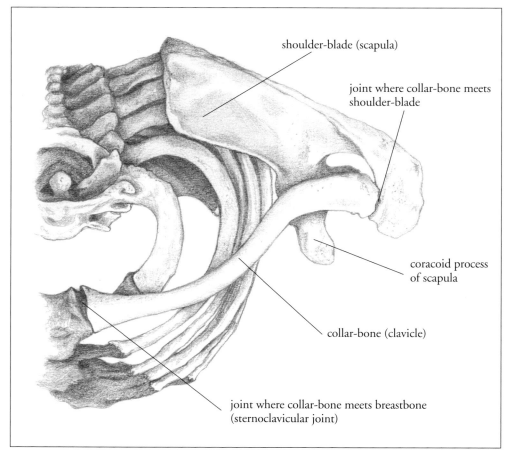

— *Fig. 43* —
Left half of shoulder girdle, from above

It is particularly necessary that the width of the shoulder girdle be maintained at moments when the hands are needed near the middle of the body. Many activities call for this – eating, for example, and typing, knitting, riding, knocking in a nail... Make your own list to suit your lifestyle – you will find it is endless. These are the moments when we are all tempted to forget that the arms are perfectly well able to get the hands where we want them, without dragging the shoulders along with them. (**Chapter 25**)

Sometimes, naturally, a shoulder-blade is obliged to accompany an arm. This is structurally unavoidable when the upper arm is lifted above shoulder height: then, the shape of the shoulder joint means that the bone in the upper arm *(humerus)* takes the shoulder-blade along for the ride – and a good thing, too. (If you want to hang by the hands from a branch, for example, it is just as well that the muscle system is reinforced by bone.) Sometimes, too, if you need to reach a long way forward, with simply no other way of getting at something, the shoulder-blade can be allowed to leave its usual place and slip forward around the side of the ribcage, to give added length to the arm. But let me emphasize that this is a last resort tactic, to be used when there is no other way: used frequently, it destroys the stability of the framework and undermines efficiency of movement. In most circumstances, the shoulder-blades should be regarded as belonging to the framework of the trunk; only rarely should they be treated as belonging to the arms. If properly treated, shoulders and their associated musculature perform strong, subtle and useful liaison work between arms and back. Shoulders, therefore, should not be asked to perform movements that can be carried out more effectively by moving the upper arm in the shoulder joint, or by changing the angle at the elbow, or both. Misuse of the shoulders can impair their usefulness for their real tasks.

Unfortunately, the possibilities of the shoulder joint are often ignored and many people displace their shoulder-blades quite regularly when doing all sorts of tasks that do not call for any such thing: cutting bread, cleaning saucepans, writing, even washing hands. If you remember that you would like to let your shoulder girdle be wide, your versatile arms can usually find alternative ways of getting your hands where you want them.

Moreover, let us not forget that the legs also can help: bending the whole trunk forward from the hip-joint can be a useful way of adding to your reach, and so indeed can a proper use of all the leg joints. (**Chapters 22, 23**)

Now that we have looked at the support for the 'tool', in the next chapter we shall consider the tool itself.

---

1. Gray's *Anatomy*, p. 318 (Osteology. The Appendicular Skeleton: Phylogeny and Functions).
2. *ibid.* p. 316.
3. See particularly the relationship of *serratus anterior* with the external oblique muscle of the abdomen.
4. Gray's *Anatomy*, p. 424 (Arthrology. Movements of the shoulder girdle).
5. *trapezius, rhomboids, latissimus dorsi.*

CHAPTER 25

THE CUTTING EDGE

The hand is the cutting edge of the mind.
J. Bronowski *The Ascent of Man*

We have seen the shoulder girdle to be the supporting structure from which the arms are suspended. Clearly, the arms themselves exist to put our hands where we want them, for the hands are the business end of this splendid piece of equipment. There is no part of us more characteristic of everything we think of as human, nothing more closely related to the human mind than the human hand.

By their capacity for both observation and action, our hands link the mind to the world around us; they are the most immediate and obvious means by which we can affect it. To do so, first and foremost they must supply us continuously with information about our surroundings – they are not only tools but antennae. In performing both functions they frequently call on the co-operation of the eyes. It is not for nothing that our arms are so arranged that we can easily bring objects to where both eyes can focus on them. Indeed, this ability is so useful that sometimes we neglect much of the information that comes to us via the sense of touch – which is a pity. Our hands, given the chance, are able to appreciate many subtleties. This seems so important that I should like forthwith to suggest a couple of experiments to you.

❏ *Experiment 1*

Just where you are, place a hand lightly on the various things within your immediate reach, one after the other. Don't grasp them – leave your hand empty, as it were, ready to receive information, that's all. Use your whole palm or just the fingertips, according to the size and shape of the object. Perhaps the first thing you notice is that some things feel warmer or cooler than others, or than your hand itself.

Now try resting your hand on each object for a moment longer: you will probably find that even when your hand is quite still it tells you something about the texture of what it is touching. This may arouse your curiosity, so now move your hand slightly.

Can you say whether more information is getting through to you from the palm or from the fingertips? Vary the pressure a bit. Do you learn more from light or firm pressure? What does your hand have to tell you about the shapes of things?

From where I sit as I type this, I can touch not only various parts of the computer, but also the polished surface of the table, its unpolished underside, several books, pen, pencil and rubber, a brass candlestick, flowers in a ceramic vase, nuts in a bowl, my glasses and the cloth for cleaning them, a packet of tissues, my own face, teeth and hair, silk blouse, woollen skirt, nylon tights – all these things feel very different, even the quality of paper in the various books. I find that a very light touch tells me most about the surface of things, the grain in the wood of the table, for example. A slightly firmer contact allows me to notice something about underlying structures, e.g. the bone in my chin announces not only its presence but how far below the surface it lies. When I place my hands around the bowl I know something about its form; if I push or lift it, even very slightly, I also get some idea of its weight.

❏ *Experiment 2*

You might look again at the same objects *without* touching them, just remembering what you know about the feel of each one. Then do the same with other things in the room, remembering or imagining what they are like to touch, pretending to yourself that you are just about to touch them. You will probably find that in most cases you have an expectation of what touching each object will be like, whereas looking at something unfamiliar in this way will awaken curiosity. Both expectation and curiosity will make your hands more alert. I have found this quite a good way of waking up my hands before playing the violin. It is certainly a useful game for people who may tend to collapse their hands and make their arms heavier than they really are.

People don't always give themselves a chance to make use of the sensitivity of their hands. I once knew a woman who had persistent pain in her arms, for no obvious reason ... until I discovered, to my surprise, that the sense of touch had very little significance for her. We were talking clothes one day, and she looked genuinely bewildered when I mentioned using touch to judge the quality of cloth, or when, admiring her new leather handbag, I revelled in the softness of its suede lining. Indeed, she insisted that she had bought her dress for no other reason than that she liked the colour, and similarly that she had chosen her handbag to go with the dress. It seemed to me that such lack of interest in how things feel to the touch was related to the pain in her arms, for I have noticed that some people suffer from being too busy or too anxious to notice what they are touching. Touch is vital to us; it is not fanciful to suggest that when the hands are not given the chance to live as antennae, the arms and shoulders can become heavy with boredom, or stiff with anxiety.

All these objects around us, all the things we use, move, examine, manipulate, we deal with by means of our hands, and in doing so we make use of what our hands are telling us about them. Experience also plays a part – we already know that roses can prick, that soap is slippery. Our hands, adapting to the present situation, are capable of combining remembered knowledge with new sensory input. This enables them to react appropriately to the needs of the moment. Truly, the hand has its 'cunning'[1]. To quote Gray's *Anatomy*:

> '... mankind goes far beyond any other creature in his endlessly variable application of manipulative skills, the hands being the responsive tools of his unrivalled mental development.'[2]

While it is true that the hands of some primates share many characteristics with our own hands, 'the human thumb ... is even better developed for opposition than in other primates.'[3]

I once knocked over a jar of marmalade while I was holding glasses in both hands. Contriving – but only just – to save the jar from falling without dropping the glasses, I felt at that moment as though instead of hands I had only paws. I began to wonder what human life would be like today, if our ancestors had never grown thumbs capable of opposing the fingers so as to hold things firmly and with precision. Without an opposable thumb and all the possibilities that it implies, I can scarcely imagine that tools or writing would have been developed – or any of the activities that derive from them. I suppose our forebears would not have begun to fashion the simple tools that enabled mankind to make more advanced tools and machinery, in which case would we now have any crafts, any industry? Without writing, exchange of information of any kind would have been limited – could science as we know it have developed? Similar questions apply to many activities that we now take for granted. What musical instruments could we make and play? What games could we amuse ourselves with, beyond such simple pleasures as kicking stones about? Whatever one calls to mind, it seems that everything in our civilisation, or in any other civilisation that we know about, depends to some extent directly or indirectly on the fact that the thumb can be opposed to the fingers.

Some creatures do remarkably skilful things – weaver birds, beavers, termites, for example – but, being unable to 'turn their hand' to the vast variety of uses we take for granted, they are compelled to remain specialists. Some exceptional people show astonishing ability in overcoming handicaps: paintings by artists who hold a brush in the mouth or between the toes show what human beings can accomplish when the mind seizes on an idea. Nevertheless, if none of us had ever had thumbs as we know them, many activities would be so difficult that the idea of them might not even have occurred to us.

To what extent thumbs evolved to meet the demands of our mental development, how much the possibilities offered by our thumbs served to stimulate our ideas, I can only speculate. But what is certain is that *the thumb lives and moves in a different field of action from the fingers* and that this difference is essential to the efficient performance of most activities of which our hands are capable. If we overlook the difference or misunderstand it, we are likely to misuse the thumb and indeed the whole hand – and so to deny ourselves some of the advantages we have as human beings.

The equipment

Let us take a look at the hand and its backup equipment, and in particular at the movements available to us for use separately or in an enormous variety of combinations. I suggest that you observe your own hands, checking my statements as you read.

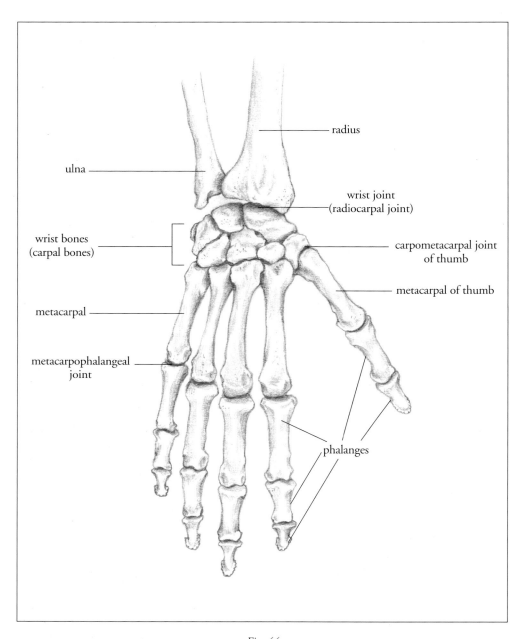

— Fig. 44 —
Bones of the hand

Fingers (fig. 44)

Three small bones *(phalanges)* go to make up a finger, and for each finger there is a fourth bone *(metacarpal)* lying within the hand and forming a link between finger and wrist. Each finger thus has three joints which can be flexed or extended with varying degrees of independence. The joints nearest to the tips of the fingers cannot usually be operated independently of the second set of joints. Note, however, that the joints furthest from the tips *(metacarpophalangeal joints)* can be flexed while the fingers are straight; they can also be extended while the other two joints are in flexion.

Counting from the tips of the fingers, on the palm side of the hand, only the first two sets of creases correspond to joints; the third set of joints, where the knuckles are, correspond more nearly to creases in the palm. The creases where the fingers meet the palm can be confusing: they show where the skin folds, but it is good to notice where the movement really occurs.

As the fingers flex, they tend to slope very slightly to meet the flexed thumb. The little finger, which has furthest to go, has an extra muscle that can actively turn (rotate) it towards the thumb.[4] Don't expect to find this muscle in the finger itself: it runs from the wrist to the metacarpal, and helps to cup the palm. (You will see it in action when we get to Experiment 3.)

Fingers can also move sideways, away from or towards each other. Total finger independence is precluded by the design, therefore attempts to impose it by force are dangerous; in any case they are sure to fail.

The thumb

The thumb has two phalanges and a metacarpal. It is at the joint where the metacarpal meets the wrist that the thumb enjoys the great freedom so crucial to human skill. *Flexion* of all or any of the three joints will point the tip of the thumb across the palm, towards the little finger; *extension* of these joints carries the tip in the opposite direction. The thumb 'lies in a plane set almost at right angles to that of the fingers'[5] and should not be placed in the same plane as the fingers unless there is a clear reason for doing so. The hand can adapt passively to a flat surface – so why prepare it by actively removing the thumb from its natural habitat? An unthinking habit of taking the thumb out of its normal sphere of action (fig. 45) can have a stiffening effect and render less readily available the function of *opposition*, which I suggest you now examine.

❑ *Experiment 3 (fig. 46)*

To recognize one of the most splendid advantages of your hand:
a) Fold the thumb loosely inside the fingers; this is *flexion*. Release the fingers to see where flexion has taken your thumb.
b) Press the *pulp* of the thumb (the flat part near the tip) against the corresponding part of the straight little finger. This is an extreme example of the all-important movement called *opposition*, in which the metacarpal and the middle section of the thumb rotate so that the thumb can oppose the fingers. (The joint nearest the tip of the thumb is not designed to twist.) Note that flexion and opposition combine in vary-

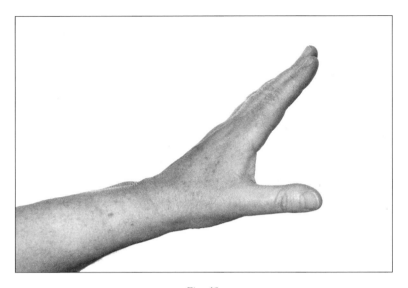

— Fig. 45a —

Thumb in its own plane

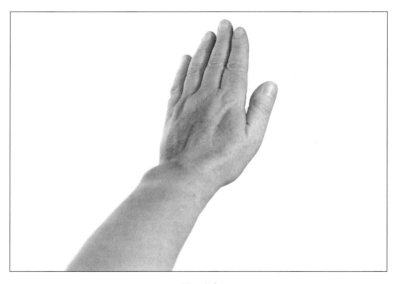

— Fig. 45b —

Thumb in fingers' plane

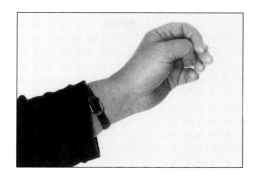 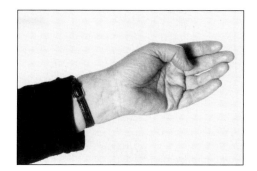

Experiment 3a) Thumb in flexion

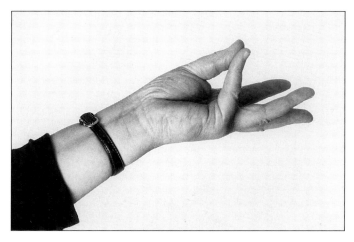

Experiment 3b) Opposition of thumb and little finger

— *Fig. 46* —

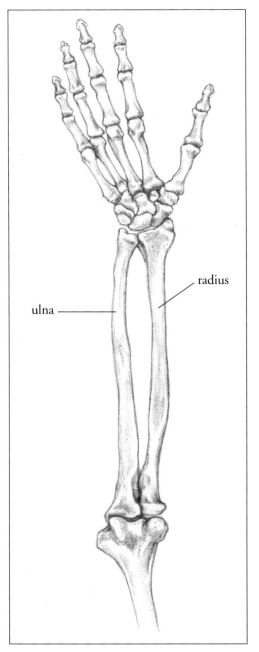

— Fig. 47 —
Right hand, palm up

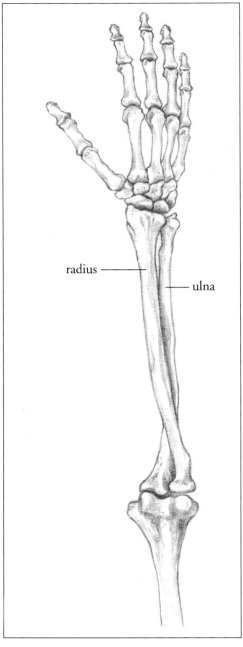

— Fig. 48 —
Right hand, palm down

ing degrees, offering many possible relationships of thumb to fingers; choice is further enlarged by the fact that the distance between thumb and palm can be increased – e.g. in order to grasp a large object. These movements blend into one another.[6]

The wrist (fig. 44)

At the wrist we have eight small bones, arranged in two rows and interlocking with each other, thanks to their shape, and joined by ligaments in such a way as to allow a limited amount of give between them. Three of them form part of the *wrist joint*[7] where the hand as a unit moves in relation to the forearm. Others articulate with the metacarpals, within the body of the hand; here again, the amount of play is limited, so far as the index, major and ring fingers are concerned. (The special possibilities of the metacarpal associated with the little finger, and the vastly greater freedom of the thumb, are described above.) Changes occur within the delicate wrist complex so as to allow for flexion, extension, and small lateral movements of the hand in relation to the forearm. Notice that these possibilities can also be used for permitting arm movements when the hand stays in the same place. (Musicians, please note that technical discussions about the 'wrist' could be clarified by stating whether it is the joint that is referred to, or the carpal bones, or whether the term is used loosely to mean the lower part of the forearm.)

The forearm

It is in the forearm (not the wrist) that we make the movements that turn the hand from the palm-up to the palm-down position and vice versa. When the palm is upward, the radius and ulna are side by side (fig. 47). To turn the palm downward, the radius, taking the hand with it, rotates on the ulna, crossing it obliquely (fig. 48). This movement is known as *pronation*. Turning the palm upward again is called *supination*. These movements, more easily seen at the wrist end of the bones than at the elbow, are sometimes mistaken for wrist movements. To make them quite clear to yourself, try them with your elbow against your side.

The elbow

With or without the rotation described above, the elbow allows flexion and extension.

The upper arm

The head of the bone of the upper arm *(humerus)* turns about in a shallow cavity in the shoulder-blade. This meeting-place is the shoulder-joint. Note where it is: perhaps further out to the side than you think. This ball-and-socket arrangement permits an enormous variety of movements, chiefly in the space in front of us and to the side; backward movements are much more limited. Rotation of the upper arm can be blended with the rotating forearm movements of pronation and supination, enhancing or varying their effect on the hand. Forearm and upper arm can also be rotated independently of each other, and even in opposite directions.

We have spoken of all these joints, all these movements, chiefly in terms of the possibilities they offer of *putting* our hands where we want them. Let us not neglect the other set of choices they offer: many of the movements described can be used passively when we want to *keep* the hands where we want them, while moving the body.

Managing the equipment

It is one thing to examine the details of our equipment, the better to appreciate its possibilities. It is another to ensure that we use these possibilities to the best advantage. There is a solution so absurdly simple that it is easily overlooked. The golden rule is: *lead with the business end.* I mean what you see when a toddler reaches for a sweet: the fingers and thumb go to the desired object, grasp it, and then make straight for the mouth – no questions asked about how. Adults could learn from this, for when the business end leads, we can normally rely on all the complicated equipment doing its job.

If there should be a problem, the first thing to ask yourself is what obstacles you may be putting in the way of smooth functioning. Are you blocking a joint that might be called on to participate? Or are you starting a movement from the wrong end of the tool – i.e. does the upper arm end get busy before the fingers and thumb have a chance to start towards their objective? The shoulder, the neck, even the head might be the culprit, for sometimes the site of interference is distant and not obvious. Pause a moment, spare some attention for the framework, then ask the business end to lead the way.

Arms and balance

It is obvious that many arm movements displace weight from within our base to outside it, and that this has an effect on balance. (**Compare this with what I have already said about balance: Chapters 13 and 21, 22, 23.**) All day long, we all move our hands about, usually somewhere in front of the body, and our arms join in. What does this do to our balance? If you balance a doll on its feet, and then move its arms forward, the doll will fall forward. So why don't we fall, too? We seldom think about this, but several solutions are possible, and some are better than others. Here are a couple of experiments that may make this clearer.

❏ *Experiment 4*

Stand facing a bookcase, about arm's length from it, ready to take a book that is about level with your shoulders. As you reach for it, something must be done about balancing the weight of your arm as it goes forward outside your base. This *could* be done by stiffening your legs, which I don't advise. More probably, you might compensate by throwing your shoulders back, tilting the ribcage and creating a 'hollow back'. However, you could allow the whole body to compensate by a tiny backward movement that makes use of your free ankles, leaving the rest of you undisturbed. In this case, the movement will be so small that you will not really have to *do* it at all: it will be enough if you just decide that it is the only balance adjustment you are going to agree to just now – it is *more a permission than an action.*

Remember, the free poise of the head (**Chapter 14**) is a factor affecting this experiment and the following one – of course, because it influences every movement.

❏ *Experiment 5*

See what happens when you are seated and need to move your arms in front of you. Even to make a small movement with elbows partly bent, it is advisable to apply the same principle as in Experiment 4 – but now it will have to be your hip-joints that are concerned, as the lowest available joint that could allow the adaptation to occur. (**See Chapter 22.**)

In this chapter we have discussed a lot of possible movements. Consider the very great number of ways in which each can be used alone, in combination, or merging into others; consider, too, the infinite variations of degree, speed, strength, lightness, weight, firmness, delicacy, fluency and meaning that can be applied to them ... and you begin to appreciate some of the ways in which the backup equipment serves your hands as they live out their two-way relationship with your mind and with your surroundings.

---

1. *O.E.D.: Cunning* Knowledge how to do a thing; ability, skill. (arch.) 'Let my right hand forget her cunning' (Psalm 137).
2. Gray's *Anatomy*, p. 558 (Myology. The movements of the hand).
3. *ibid.* p. 318 (Osteology).
4. *opponens digiti minimi.*
5. Gray's *Anatomy*, p. 399 (Arthrology. The movements and mechanisms of joints).
6. I have avoided naming thumb movements in the main text, because of divergent terminology. In Gray's terms (pp. 439 and 555–6) flexion merges with opposition, and the two can blend with abduction; extension ultimately turns into lateral rotation; adduction draws the thumb alongside the index. Gray's makes clear the thumb's special field of activity. (Kapandji uses the same terms, but with different meanings, except in the case of opposition.) It seems to me that the resources of the human hand defy complete description – and can best be appreciated by those who make the most subtle use of them. (I have known the drawing of a pianist's hand in Kapandji (vol. 1, p. 175) to evoke derision in pianists – and in fact those pianists I have observed are manifestly correct in denying that they would normally approach a key in the way indicated.)
7. the radio-carpal joint.

CHAPTER 26

MORE ABOUT HANDS

> Unless we live what we know, we do not even know it. It is
> only by making our knowledge part of ourselves, through
> activity, that we enter into the reality that is signified by
> our concepts.
>
> Thomas Merton *Thoughts in Solitude*

Here are a few more experiments designed to draw your attention to your privileged position as the owner of a pair of human hands – and to help you to notice some fundamental factors that apply to everything you do with them.

❏ *Experiment 1*

Let one arm hang by your side, the fingers and thumb doing absolutely nothing. With the upper arm still touching your side, gently flex the elbow so that it forms roughly a right angle – still doing nothing with the hand. The thumb and index finger will now be uppermost, the little finger nearest the floor. If you really do nothing with your wrist, your hand will be hanging so that the little finger side of it seems to be dropping away from the forearm a bit *(ulnar deviation)*: that is, the metacarpal of the thumb is more or less in line with the forearm (fig. 49). With elbow flexed as described, this is the starting point for all the other experiments in this chapter. It is an attitude of neutral readiness – let us call it NR for short.

It often happens that when the idea comes to them to perform even a straightforward task with their hands, people start by making unnecessary efforts, such as locking the elbows, or lifting the shoulders, or flexing the wrists, or moving the thumb in ways that reduce its availability for appropriate action. Some, possibly wanting to prove to themselves how 'relaxed' they are when their hands have nothing special to do for the moment, seem to collapse their wrists in gestures that involve extreme flexion. NR avoids both of these traps: it is the attitude from which you can most easily move into whatever you want your hands to do – so don't be in a hurry to change it.

183

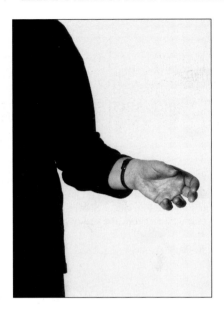

— *Fig. 49* —
Experiment 1) neutral readiness

❏ *Experiment 2*

Start in NR, and this time, without changing the angle between forearm and upper arm, move your elbow slightly forward from its resting place. This is a movement of the upper arm, the top of which can move in the shoulder-joint without disturbing the shoulder itself. If you did nothing but that, your hand is now higher than it was at the start. Leave the upper arm where it is and let your elbow open so that your forearm is roughly horizontal again. Try combining these two movements so as to reach for something just in front of your hand. Many people, when they do this, lock either elbow or shoulder-joint or both, and get involved in something less convenient and more complicated, so this is well worth investigating.

❏ *Experiment 3*

Start in NR. Still leaving your hand severely alone, turn your forearm gently so that your palm faces upward. Let the weight of your hand take your wrist into slight extension (if it wasn't already). With your other hand, place various small objects on your palm, without moving thumb or fingers. You might try this with a matchbox or a pencil, with peanuts or smarties or your loose change. Better still, ask a friend to put the things in your hand, and to help you to notice if your thumb reacts unnecessarily. If you can accept things in the cup of your hand, and not feel the slightest need to do anything about it, you have begun to know your hand in what I call its *receptive mode* (fig. 50).

184

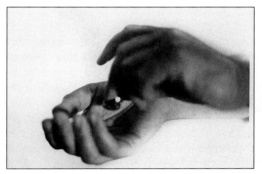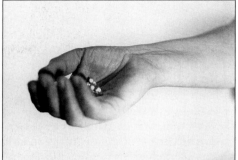

— Fig. 50 —
Experiment 3) receptive mode

❏ *Experiment 4*

Start by repeating Experiment 3, and now go on to play with combining the receptive mode with movements of upper arm and forearm, as in Experiment 2. Then see if, leaving your elbow at your side, you can move your hand across your body, then out to the side, without needing to close your hand to save the smarties or whatever. (This calls for a movement of the *humerus* in the shoulder-joint.) You could also repeat the experiment, placing something slightly heavier in your hand (a small ornament, perhaps) noticing how easily you adapt to the change in weight. Note also that the hands can often be in receptive mode when carrying large and even heavy objects, where the hands' task is chiefly one of adaptation to the shape of the object – a punch-bowl, for example – as strength and lifting power can be provided for elsewhere in the body.

❏ *Experiment 5*

Repeat Experiment 4, to the point where your palm is upward, wrist in slight extension. Let thumb meet index as if taking a pinch of salt. Elbow still at your side, and *without disturbing the hand/forearm relationship*, turn the forearm gently so that the palm faces down. I think you will still find that the thumb is nearly continuous with the forearm, the wrist in slight extension. The fact that the hand is not busy does not mean that it should flop from a flexed wrist; nor does the fact that the hand is not all floppy mean that the wrist is stiff. Both hand and wrist are free enough and lively enough to be available for movement. If you are using your framework as I have described throughout, the whole body will be contributing to the support of hand and arm. These moving parts will not now need to stiffen to support themselves. (That is how people hurt themselves.)

❏ *Experiment 6*

Combine Experiments 5 and 2.

185

❏ *Experiment 7*

Combine Experiment 6 with lifting and lowering the elbow sideways, by means of a movement of the upper arm in the shoulder-joint. What difference does this make to where your fingers arrive?

If you spend a lot of time at the keyboard of a computer or typewriter, Experiments 5–7 are particularly important for you. Without good forearm pronation, you would have to disorganize your shoulders in order to get your hands the right way up. This is the start of a vicious spiral, since people who have a habit of misusing their shoulders cannot achieve proper forearm pronation: what they often have is **pain**, somewhere in the neck/shoulder/arm/hand complex. If freedom of forearm rotation is unduly limited or presents difficulties for you, do not try to force it. You would do better to spend some time and thought on the behaviour of your shoulders and of your thumbs. (**See also** Chapter 30.)

Holding, wielding, carrying, lifting

We have five main ways of holding objects:
1) we can use our hands in their receptive mode, as described above. Typical use: carrying a large punch bowl – the hands remain passive while making contact with the object, then they do just enough work to maintain firm contact while receiving its weight. Other choices:
2) the power grip;
3) the precision grip;
4) the pincer grip;
5) the hook grip.

The power grip *(fig. 51)*

Typical use: wielding a hammer. This is the grip we use when something has to be held firmly in the palm of the hand, with the fingers flexed around the object and the thumb supplying counter-pressure.

People who do aikido know that if the wrist of an opponent can be put into extreme flexion his grip will be weakened because the thumb can no longer oppose the fingers effectively. Let me point out a corollary: to hold something firmly, the most effective way is to approach the object in such a way that your thumb continues the line of the forearm. Your wrist will thus be in slight *extension* and slightly turned towards the little finger side *(ulnar deviation)* – two conditions that favour a firm grip without unnecessary strain. The grip will be further improved if the hand is really open to start with, i.e. if, without flexing the wrist, you extend all the joints of fingers and thumb just before grasping the object. With the object well and truly in the palm of the hand, the still-lengthening fingers and thumb can *then* wrap around the object in such a way that muscles are at an even greater advantage in maintaining the grip. The more efficient the grip, the more readily available will be the movements of forearm and upper arm necessary for carrying out the desired activity.

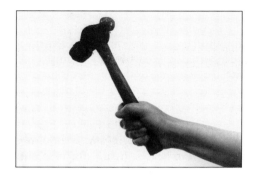

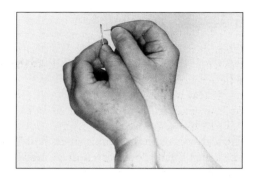

— Fig. 51 —
Power grip

— Fig. 52 —
Precision grip

❏ *Experiment 8*

Take a fairly substantial magazine and roll it up tightly. Grip it firmly, then ask someone to try and take it away from you. Did you open your hand (as described above) before you grasped the magazine? Do it the other way – what difference did it make?

The precision grip (fig. 52)

Typical use: picking up a pin, pencil, or small tool. This grip is used for holding small objects between the tips of the thumb and one or more fingers. Thumb and fingers will then be ready to co-operate in movements of flexion and extension so as to manipulate the object. In this they can count on the co-operation of all the rest of the backup equipment, always provided that the rest of the limb is available for use. Problems arise when the owner is so absorbed in a tricky job for fingers and thumb that other joints are allowed to become fixed just when they might be needed for small adaptations. Notice that we sometimes use a combination of precision and power grips in the same hand: e.g. thumb and index manipulating something that the other fingers are holding steady.

It is important to note that the precision grip, like the power grip, is most efficient when *the thumb prolongs the line of the forearm*, i.e. when the wrist is in slight extension and slight ulnar deviation. Even when no gripping is involved, *this is a natural attitude of the hand, favouring finger agility without straining the wrist.* N.B. This is intended to indicate a basis for healthy behaviour for a hand at work: it is not to be taken as recommending any fixed position, for the hands are always in the process of making small adaptations to the needs of the moment.

❏ *Experiment 9*

Flex the wrists, and thread a needle while maintaining wrist flexion. Then thread a needle, using finger and thumb movements while steadying wrists lightly against each other (i.e. the wrists are in extension). Compare the two methods for precision and comfort.

The pincer grip *(fig. 53)*

Typical use: reading a newspaper. For this grip the fingers are straight and the thumb, opposing them, comes as near to the finger-tips as it can reach. Again, for ease and comfort, the thumb will almost certainly need to be more or less in line with the fore-arm. If you tend to over-flex your fingers or to clench your fists for no particular reason, you might try playing, lightly and easily, with pincer-type movements. I think you will find them rather healthy for your hands.

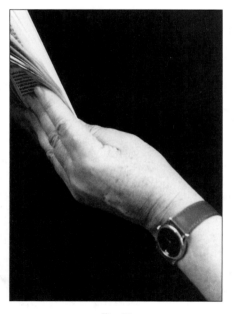

— *Fig. 53* —

Pincer grip: flexion of the fingers occurs only
at the metacarpophalangeal joints.

The hook grip *(fig. 54)*

Typical use: carrying a suitcase. The first two phalanges are flexed, making a hook. When possible, this way of carrying is preferable to making a fist round the handle, as the weight is distributed in a more healthy way. (The thumb can be used from time to time, for guiding the load.)

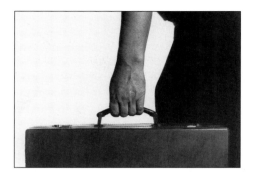 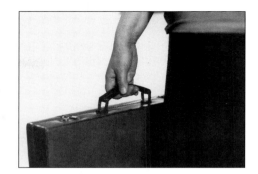

— *Fig. 54* —
Hook grip

Essential safety rules for lifting heavy objects

1) Stand as near as possible to the weight.
2) Do not pull your head backwards.
3) Keep the back long and 'in one piece' – i.e. do not bend at the waist (neither forward nor backward).
4) Do not lift the heels. If you need to get down to the weight, use the hinges at hip, knee and ankle, and slope forward like a monkey, back straight and heels on the ground. (**See Chapters 22, 23.**)
5) Do not let the shoulders flop forward. Don't go to the other extreme and pull them back! Just think of maintaining the total width of the shoulder girdle. (**See Chapter 24.**)
   Whenever there is any lifting to be done, it is most important to think first about the co-ordinated framework. If you have worked carefully through the book so far, and are really familiar with the advice given about head balance, about the shoulder girdle and about the proper relationship of legs to back, your attention to these matters should ensure that weight is accepted in a way that does not place too much strain on vulnerable parts of the structure. Having offered yourself enough time to think of these things, so as to prepare the framework to meet the demands you are about to place on it, *do not abandon all your preparations at the moment you decide to go into action.* Keep them all going as you act fairly swiftly: speed overcomes inertia. **Above all, don't pull your head backwards when things get difficult.** If you can't lift the weight without that, you probably can't lift it anyway – and will only hurt yourself if you insist on trying. Instead, remembering the same principles, push, turn or roll the weight – or get help.

It is not always easy, when faced with a difficulty, to remember good intentions and sensible precautions. That is why I so often suggest experimenting and practising on something easy, relating it to the rest of what you have understood. If we don't make a point of stopping and choosing how we are going to do things, old habits (**see Chapter 32**) have a way of deciding for us – sometimes with unfortunate consequences.

PART VI
HELPS AND HINDRANCES

CHAPTER 27

TOUCH

I hold a spade in my empty hand.
Zen koan

In Chapters 25 and 26, we discussed some of the ways in which we use that wonderful tool, the human hand. Another aspect deserves a chapter to itself: the use of the hand as a means of communication through touch. Not only in lovers' caresses and in the entire mother-baby relationship, but also in friendly hugs and backslappings, in routine handshakes, in helping sick or elderly people, even in indicating that we are trying to pass somebody in a crowded room – in all these situations, and many more, there arise moments when one's own state is directly and immediately communicated to another human being. This seems to me quite a responsibility. To accept it adequately, we need to pay attention to how we use ourselves, for thus we reduce the risk of intruding willy-nilly upon other people, of burdening them inadvertently with problems that need not concern them.

I can best explain this with a few real-life illustrations. One incident was related to me independently by two friends of mine, who also knew each other – let's call them Jean and Mary.

Jean's version: *I'm worried about Mary. I saw her in the lane, sitting on the wall, looking quite ill, so I touched her shoulder gently, and asked 'whatever is the matter?' But she shook me off, saying 'Leave me alone!' Is she heading for a breakdown or something?*

The next day I heard Mary's version: *I felt so dreadful on my way home from work yesterday that walking up the hill I had to sit down on the wall. The last straw was that Jean came along and leant on me so heavily that I thought I was going to faint. I'm afraid I may have been a bit rude to her.*

I could guess what had happened. I knew Jean as a kind person; I knew, too, that she always seemed a bit collapsed. I think that probably her hand, gentle though it may have been, communicated her own fundamental heaviness to Mary, who, already rather unwell, found it literally too much to bear.

Another example: a shoulder was recovering nicely from a sports injury when its owner, absorbed in her work, did not reply at once to a colleague's question, so he tapped her on the shoulder. Who could complain of such a thing? Nevertheless, impatience had given his touch such an aggressive quality that her shoulder sent waves of pain throughout her body for some hours. Hearing about this brought back sad memories of my mother-in-law, profoundly upset, in her last weeks, by the impatience she had felt in the hands of a (doubtless overworked) nurse. Despite the best of intentions, we do not always recognize how our current mood can affect our touch, which will nevertheless often tell others more than we would wish them to know about how we are managing ourselves, our own co-ordination, our own emotions. Such unintentional betrayals of oneself (particularly distressing to children and to elderly people unable to defend themselves) can often be avoided by taking thought to the proper management of one's own framework.

A pleasanter example is a memory I have of a mountain walk, when one of my students held out a hand in case I needed help in crossing an icy patch. At such moments, some people's touch can make one nervous, but in this case, although our hands barely made contact, I received a vivid and reassuring impression that adequate support was available if needed. The student had reached a high standard of co-ordination, clearly perceptible through the unpremeditated polite gesture.

These or similar incidents might arise casually at any moment. But some situations call for particular awareness of the need to organize one's own movements as well as possible. Anyone who uses any kind of physical technique for helping other people should be particularly sensitive to this fact. Experience and observation have convinced me that there are absolutely no massage techniques or manipulative procedures that can be guaranteed useful or even harmless, independently of the personal co-ordination of the person employing them.

The truth of this was brought home to me many years ago, when, as a relatively inexperienced Alexander teacher, I was working with a charming and courageous elderly woman whose shoulder had undergone surgery. The operation had been successful, the postoperative treatment manifestly less so, for after nearly two years she still could barely lift her hand to her mouth. Working with great care, I found I could help her to obtain a progressively greater degree of movement in the shoulder joint, and that this did not hurt her, provided that, as I gently guided her arm, I thought unceasingly about my own co-ordination as well as hers – but if my concentration flickered for a moment, she was at once in pain.

This experience made me realize, more clearly than ever, the value of my Alexander training, with its constant insistence that the primary requirement of an Alexander teacher is proper use of oneself. (See Chapter 34.) Of course, not everyone can have concentrated training of the kind we received during those three years, but surely nobody can afford to ignore the significance of touch. My training showed me, and I continue to learn, that though touch can be refined almost infinitely, there is essentially nothing esoteric about it. Just as a young child will spontaneously make itself light if it wants you to lift it, or unbelievably heavy if it is in a tantrum, so adults, too, make themselves light or heavy, and thus modify the effect they have on those they happen to touch. And even though adult life is subject to all sorts of influences that may lead us to make ourselves heavy and careless, it still seems quite natural for people to become light and sensitive when dealing with babies or small animals. To extend a similar degree of respect towards other adults does not seem a big or difficult step – it just needs thinking about.

CHAPTER 28

MORE HELP FOR YOUR BACK

... strive for repose but by means of the equilibrium
and not of the cessation of your activity.
Schiller

Much of this book has been concerned with exploring the fact that a natural good use of
oneself often emerges quite easily, provided fundamental misunderstandings can be
eliminated. Now we are going to discover a simple procedure which can be of tremendous benefit to virtually everybody. This procedure, if followed faithfully and regularly,
not only confirms and encourages good use: it gently unravels the harmful effects of
mistakes. Let me strongly urge you to try it, attending carefully to the details – though
simple, they are important.

The procedure consists, in essence, of lying on your back on the floor (not the bed)
with your head on some books (not cushions) which must not touch your neck; your
feet are on the ground, your knees bent and pointing straight upwards. (You may have
heard of this before, or have read something about it; most unfortunately, some published descriptions are incomplete, while some others are seriously misleading.) Detailed
instructions are given later in this chapter.

How, you will want to know, can such a very ordinary procedure benefit my back?
The answer is, by giving your entire framework repeated opportunities to return to the
best shape of which it is capable at a given moment. Most of us, as we go through a normal day, make some slightly awkward adaptations to the needs of balancing ourselves.
Clearly, lying down removes the balance problem; to lie down, in the way I shall describe, also invites the help of gravity in ironing out the complications in which we have
almost certainly involved ourselves. It helps to restore the equilibrium between the work
of different groups of muscles, thus helping to establish proper relationships between
the various skeletal components.

The primary and secondary curves of the spine are weight-bearing – they are supposed to be there, but if they become exaggerated, the whole structure is shortened and
muscles can no longer be maintained at an efficient working length. When you lie in the
attitude described above, subtle changes begin to occur. Lying on a firm surface, with a

firm support under your head, enhances the effect of gravity on those parts of you that are not directly supported; this tends to reduce the curves in the spine, making you a bit longer. As you know, there are muscles that normally work to support you when you are upright. (Not all of them belong directly to the spine; they are all over the place.) Some of these muscles, having been overworking, will now gradually recognize that they are at liberty to adapt to the changing situation – so you become not only longer, but wider and perhaps slightly flatter.

This subtle interplay of natural forces and the body's own wisdom requires no pushing along from you. Forget about trying to flatten your back, forget about trying to relax. If you do *nothing* about all that, you will be giving your body a chance to restore its own balances. Perhaps you will not *feel* anything happening, but this does not mean that nothing *is* happening – only that the changes occur gently and without fuss, at your body's own speed. If you have put yourself on the floor in the proper way, you have done your part. I don't advise thinking about what should be happening, or what you plan to do next. Just accept the fact that gravity is working for you now; your job is to let it get on with it. It's rather as if, having sorted your laundry, you let the machine get on with the washing.

You will need

a bit of *floor space*,
a *blanket*,
a small pile of *books*,
a piece of *thin plastic foam*.
Add *five minutes* of your time and you have the ingredients for doing yourself a lot of good.

The floor space should allow you enough room to lie down on your back with your knees bent, and to roll sideways in order to get up again. Choose somewhere out of the way of draughts and where people won't trip over you. Wrap your books and foam in the blanket and keep them handy. Shove the whole lot in a small bag and take it with you when you go away.

The blanket is for lying on, so you will not want a fluffy one. A fair-sized car rug would be suitable. *The books* are to rest your head on, so they had better not be hardbacks. (I was given some old copies of *Reader's Digest*, which are ideal, but paperbacks or telephone directories will also do nicely.) Whatever you use, *the height is of paramount importance*; and the right height varies a lot from person to person.

To judge the height of the books, sit as you normally do, and ask a friend to place his or her elbow just below your shoulder-blades, at the point of maximum outward curve. With forearm and hand forming a straight, vertical line, your friend now moves her arm straight upwards until her hand is somewhere behind your head. She then takes the books in her other hand to see how many will fit in between her hand and your head. While this is going on, you must be very sure not to move your head backwards; let it drop into neutral (as described in Chapter 14) and *never mind if this makes you look down*. To these books, add a few more, another good inch or so of thickness; you will then have the *approximate* height of the books on which you are going to rest your head. The *precise* height of books needed will probably vary from time to time, so be sure always to have a few extra to hand. Don't be astonished if you find yourself changing. Sometimes you are more tired than you think you are, sometimes better than you feel. *If in doubt, use more books rather than less:* you will know if you have too many (your chin will press on your Adam's apple). Too few, and the benefit is lost.

The thin plastic foam (from DIY shops) is so that your feet don't slip. Get a piece about two foot square (60 x 60 cm). An excellent alternative is the mesh they sell in carpet shops to stop rugs from slipping.

The time is up to you to find. The ideal would be to do this lying-down procedure for five minutes after breakfast, five minutes at lunch-time, the same at the start of the evening, and again just before going to bed. If you have any problem with your back, this is the minimum time that you really ought to spend on it – though for some people the midday time will be difficult. But whatever the difficulties, most people will admit, if pressed, that they can somehow manage to spare five minutes for themselves, a couple of times during each twenty-four hours, if they really try.

Optional extras. Some people have a little bump on the back of the head and so like to put a small piece of foam on the top of the books, If you wear jeans, you may find that the seams are uncomfortable to lie on: a small piece of foam tucked inside your jeans will help. If your back is very sore, so that lying on a hard surface is really difficult, a thicker piece of foam, running the whole length of your back, is helpful. Are you built with a ribcage that is particularly deep from front to back, so that your arms are as it were falling behind you when you are lying on your back? You may like to place a small thin cushion under the point of each elbow. This can also be a useful idea if you are very 'round-shouldered'. First work out the right place for the cushions, then don't fiddle with them once you are lying down.

How to start

Much depends on the way you get into position. It isn't difficult; with this description, you can check on details. The best way to start, I find, is as follows.

1) Spread your blanket on the floor, placing books and foam where you expect your head and feet to be when you are lying on your back with bent knees. Turn the books so that all their spines lie at the end furthest from your feet – you will not be very comfortable otherwise.

2) Stand with your feet on the foam.

3) Sit on the blanket, then get your seat as close to your feet as you can manage without straining. (It won't seem too close when you are lying down.) Hugging your knees makes it easier to place your feet, and helps you to keep your balance.

4) Allow the head to fall forwards, providing a counterweight to the trunk which is, of course, somewhat behind its base.

5) Place the feet a little way apart, at roughly the width of the hips, keeping the soles of the feet in contact with the ground.

6) Prop yourself up by putting your hands on the ground, *slightly* behind your seat,

fingers pointing out to the side.

7) Still supporting yourself on your hands, straighten your arms, keeping the shoulders wide, so that they don't get pulled up around your neck.

8) Releasing the hip-joints, allow the abdomen to fall backwards, then quickly let your arms bend, so that you are now supported on the elbows.

9) Do not linger in this position, but slide your elbows forward, so that your shoulders can continue undisturbed as your head comes to rest on the books. *NB Don't straighten your legs as you do this.*

10) If the books touch your neck, gently push them a little further away, *without lifting your head* – in this position, there is no way of lifting your head without shortening yourself. (Of course, if you misjudge things and miss the books altogether, or find them somewhere in your back, there is nothing for it but to begin again. You will soon get used to arranging things.)

11) If the books are definitely too high, use one hand on the crown of your head to lift it, while the other hand removes the top book. Repeat if necessary – you see why thin books are best. Use the same method if you need to add books.

12) If your feet are too far away, gently move them – if this is unnecessary, so much the better; hence suggestion 3) above.

13) Let your hands rest on the hip-bones, or on the floor, but preferably not on your chest or abdomen.

14) If your knees are not pointing straight up to the ceiling, move them till they are – now they will be easy to balance and you have nothing left to bother about.

Note that although it takes quite a lot of words to describe this way of getting into position, it is best to do it quite quickly and easily. So, first understand what you are going to do, and then do it without any fuss – being too careful could stiffen you.

There are advantages to the way of lying down that I have described; however, if it presents serious difficulties for you, just get there as easily as you can. This arrangement allows all sorts of good things to happen. Just be there and it will do some good. All you are responsible for is seeing to it that your knees continue to point directly upwards; if you let your legs fall out of balance, you will have extra work supporting them, so don't go to sleep! That apart, there is no need to do anything about anything; any sort of fidget is counter-productive, so don't waste time trying to improve the way you are lying. If you are seriously uncomfortable, start again; if not, just accept yourself as you are.

Getting up again. It is essential to roll over sideways. *Don't do a sit-up*, or you will undo the good you have done yourself. Plan the way you mean to roll, then do it without slowing it down too much – it's usually easier. Suppose you choose to roll to the left:

1) With your right eye, look towards your left shoulder, allowing your head to turn to the left (**see Chapter 16**).

2) Keeping knees bent, let your legs fall to the left, simultaneously passing your right hand across your body to the left.

3) A little pressure of your right hand and your left elbow against the floor and you are on all fours. From here, unless you have time for a little crawling (**Chapter 20**) you can get up, *first reminding yourself not to pull your head backwards.*

Don't stay on the floor too long; five minutes will do, or ten for a treat. It is interesting and valuable to see if you can stay awake and alert while doing nothing – cats can manage it. Little and often is what brings results – so I always beg people to stick to it, for I have seen people transformed by doing it regularly. (One man, asked if he was persevering, looked offended and said 'I am not a fool – it has helped me so much, of course I shall do it for the rest of my life.') It is not only your back that will be helped – just about every part of you will benefit. It would be a pity not to do such a simple thing that helps so much.

I do understand that many people, even when they have time, are self-conscious about doing something slightly unusual when friends or colleagues may see them. But there are people who, faithful to the procedure described above, are prepared to brave a few raised eyebrows in the cause of common sense – and I respect them for it. I have before me an account of a report to the Government which states that in Britain, back pain accounts for more than 100 million lost working days each year; back sufferers who have been off for two years are said to be unlikely to get back to work.[1] The National Back Pain Association figures give the yearly cost to the National Health Service as about £480 million, and the cost to industry, in lost production, as at least £5.1 billion. N.P.B.A. statistics also show British schoolchildren to be increasingly at risk. And in Belgium, a Ministry of Education report states that six out of ten 14-year-olds suffer from back problems.[2] I could go on and on. Given a social problem of this magnitude, anyone who takes sensible steps to avoid becoming part of the problem deserves thanks all round; and facilities for lying down during a lunch break would be worth a lot of official reports.

---

1. *The Independent*, 14th June, 1995.
2. *The Bulletin – the newsweekly of the capital of Europe*, Brussels, 21st November, 1996.

CHAPTER 29

CHAIRS AND OTHER EQUIPMENT

Stretched on the rack of a too easy chair...
Alexander Pope

Some things are so wrong that even their opposite is not right.
Karl Kraus

This book is, of course, primarily about people rather than things, and people, as we know, are highly adaptable – it is one reason for our success as a species. However, part of this adaptability surely consists in being able to avoid things that work against us, so it is worth taking a look at some of the basic equipment with which we surround ourselves, and how it affects the way we use our *human* equipment.

When we are not moving around, or standing preparatory to moving somewhere, we often like to sit or lie down, and in response to this wish, we have invented various objects. I have never quite understood the degree to which *chairs* are held to blame for our muscular and skeletal problems. 'Of course,' people are heard to say, 'chairs are unnatural' – as though that explained a lot of things. But is it true that there is something unnatural about chairs? Granted that in warm dry weather our primitive forebears must have felt it natural to sit or squat wherever they happened to find themselves, in a northern climate there were presumably plenty of occasions when a fallen tree or a handy rock would have been preferable to wet, muddy ground. Nor can it really be argued that there is something unnatural about sitting in itself. The joints that allow squatting (which is indisputably 'natural') also allow us to perform the interrupted squat known as sitting. Chairs *as such* are not the villains they have been made out to be.

I think, however, that there is something seriously wrong in our attitude to the whole business of being seated, and that this results sometimes in choosing quite unsuitable chairs for our purposes, and sometimes in misusing chairs that may be all right in themselves. Suppose we ask ourselves *why we sit* in the first place, and what kind of chairs we need for different purposes. Essentially, I suppose we may say that there are chairs for working and chairs for resting.

Work chairs (also for eating, and for sitting down for just a moment)

Sometimes we sit so as to be conveniently placed for doing some kind of work with hands or feet, or both; or sometimes just in order to rest the feet and legs, or to give the back a change of work. All this is surely reasonable, since the seat-bones, ideal for sitting on, allow the expanding framework of the body to be balanced in a variety of attitudes, according to what we are doing. (See Chapter 23.)

Seats for work chairs

The best seats for this type of use are *firm, flat and horizontal*, permitting maximum efficiency of balance, combined with maximum freedom of arm and leg movements. Chairs with shaped seats are undesirable; so are those that have ridges on the edge of the seat. A thin layer of padding is acceptable, but seats that are really soft are tiring, because, instead of supporting you, they oblige *you* to adapt to them all the time.

Chair seats that do damage

The most disastrous chairs that I have seen so far are those stacking chairs consisting of a tubular metal frame with a canvas seat and back: not only do they give no support, but the metal parts prevent any reasonable placing of the user's thighs. Almost as damaging (whatever the material) are *any* chairs with seats higher in front than at the back. They are to be seen everywhere, but I think they first became popular purely for convenience of stacking, without regard to the comfort or health of the user. *No amount of 'physical education' will undo the damage done to schoolchildren condemned to spend hours of every day sitting on such chairs. Good chairs can never guarantee good sitting, but it is scandalous that children, forced to use chairs on which it is impossible to sit properly, are thus moulded for a future of poor co-ordination, back pain, and other health problems.*

Forward-sloping seats are sometimes advocated – and I daresay they make a nice change from being forced backwards whether you like it or not. But the forward slope encourages feet and legs to be constantly busy to stop you slipping forwards. This disadvantage may pass unnoticed by the many people who habitually overwork their legs anyway, but the underlying problem – misuse of legs and back – has still not been addressed. The legs tend to become disproportionately active, to the detriment of the back, and ultimately of the legs themselves. Some very tall people like these chairs, but anyone who has acquired proper balanced sitting will not have difficulty in adapting to any *horizontal* seat of whatever height, provided the feet can be on the floor. (See Chapters 21–2–3.)

Backs for work chairs

On any seat that does not allow you to balance properly, you will tend to collapse at the waist, rounding the lumbar spine; this is bad for your back (and for other parts of you). A chair back that pushes your lower back in again does not correct this fault; it compounds it, for in fact you will only be collapsing in the opposite direction. (See chapter 8.) Only when *seats* are adequate does it become possible to discuss chair *backs*. If you are sitting in good balance, and provided you know the proper way of compensating for arm movements (**Chapter 25, experiments 4 and 5**) you will probably not really need a back to your chair as long as you have something interesting to do. (I don't suppose you usually lean back in your chair when you are eating!) The times you will want a back-rest of some kind are the moments when you pause for thought or have to wait for something. Sometimes, too, when one is tired – and inclined to make oneself more so by shrinking and collapsing – it can be nice if the chair invites one to expand again.

A sensible backrest will touch you behind the shoulder-blades, or *very slightly* below them; you should be able to come into contact with it by letting yourself slope back slightly, in one piece, *from the hip-joints*. This means, of course, that the seat should not be too deep from front to back; if it is, you will either collapse or stiffen before you arrive at your backrest, or else you will have too much pressure on your thighs (bad for circulation). If you haven't collapsed, you won't need a large area of contact; a backrest with a flattish surface is better than a rounded one.

Work chairs – a suggestion

In my experience, it is best when chairs are not too elaborate; trying to make everything fit perfectly can create problems. My favourite working chair is one I bought in a village junk shop: it looks like a child's drawing and is suitable for all the adult pupils I have met so far. (The woman in figs. 37 and 40 is sitting on it.) When inventing chairs for people who have to spend long hours at a desk or workbench, designers might do worse than to take as a starting point a good piano stool. To do the work of a pianist – skilled as it is, and physically demanding, too – it is essential to be comfortably and reliably seated, for the hands must command a wide area, while the movements of the feet on the pedals have to be co-ordinated with those of the hands. Therefore, in every good concert hall you will find stable stools with *horizontal* seats, very firmly padded with horsehair covered in leather (less sweaty than plastic); the padding is quilted to keep it from shifting. These stools, of adjustable height, are expensive but extremely durable. I don't see why they couldn't be adapted, for more general use, by the addition of a backrest such as I have described. (Castors could be added when necessary.) In the most exacting conditions, the best piano stools have proved their suitability for generations of pianists – who, like the rest of us, come in all shapes and sizes. Surely designers of chairs might learn from all this experience?

Chairs for rest

Here there is more scope for variation, but the principle still holds that a chair cannot be good if it forces you to collapse. Why do people want to collapse, anyway? If you are merely *rather* tired, a more balanced way of sitting will refresh you; if your tiredness is unbearable, lying down is what you need. Very low, over-soft 'easy' chairs and sofas are an abomination: most people can hardly get into or out of them without doing themselves harm – and what happens in between hardly bears thinking of.

Flopping about in a collapsed state is really harmful. I remember an evening when I dropped in on some friends, to find one of them half-lying most uncomfortably on a soggy sofa, complaining of acute back pain. In a corner was a well-made old-fashioned dining-room chair with arms. I persuaded him to sit on that instead, and – since he had recently started Alexander lessons – reminded him of a few basic principles. He had begun to feel much better, when his wife, returning with coffee, said, 'Goodness, doesn't he look silly sitting up there!' Rather peeved, I retorted, 'Not half so silly as he looked on that sofa, suffering when there was a simple solution.' I know it can be a bit difficult to choose a firm chair or stool, but if you can resist well-meant invitations to 'sit here and be comfortable', I think you will find it is worth it, particularly if your back tends to give problems.

There are many types of resting chair that are reasonable and do no harm. High-backed wing-chairs can be very comfortable, if the seat is firm and not too deep from front to back. The ideal depth, of course, depends on the length of your thighs – you don't want to have to collapse at the waist in order to reach the back of the chair. I have seen a modern chair in padded leather that I should love to have: sitting in it, one leans slightly backwards, which in this case is all right, because the attitude – head against the high back and feet on a large matching footstool – feels luxuriously restful but does not distort you. My pet chair for watching television is a little antique nursing chair, very low with a small padded seat and nearly straight back. And on a chaise-longue – and some modern equivalents – you can put your feet up while still taking part in whatever is going on.

Kneeling chairs

Sometimes people ask my opinion of the type of chair where you kneel rather than keeping your feet on the floor. These chairs are widely publicized as correcting faulty posture, because you can hardly keep your balance if you slump. Unfortunately, anyone with a tendency to slump will probably hollow the lower back instead, *as depicted in the advertisements (!)* – and this is not really an improvement, it is only what has been called 'a different sort of badly'. (See Chapters 8 and 23.) There can also be problems if the pressure comes on the wrong part of the knee. (In fairness I must say that I have known one person for whom such a chair was suitable for a particular purpose, and who could use it thanks to a back that was already in unusually good condition.)

Fun chairs

Rocking-chairs are fun, and so are the big inflatable balls that children enjoy bouncing around on. But both, if used all day, will encourage perpetual fidgeting and over-use of leg muscles. For amusement, why not? An alternative to sensible work chairs? Certainly not.

Role of the feet in sitting

I often notice that people are so uncomfortable on the chairs they have either chosen or had wished on them that they make things even worse by doing strange things with their feet and legs. If the feet are comfortably in contact with the floor, balance is facilitated, and a lot of useful information is received and used by the rest of the body. When the feet are tucked up under the chair, with only the toes in contact with the floor, a great deal of unnecessary tension is created in the legs, all the way up to the hips, and the back has correspondingly less chance of arranging itself well. From time to time, of course, one moves just for the sake of changing position for a moment, so I would never say 'never', but crossing one knee over the other is not a frightfully good habit: indulged in too often, it creates problems around the hip-joints, and encourages the back to collapse at waist level. On the other hand, crossing the ankles (fig. 40) can be a useful compromise for women in short skirts, because the knees are kept fairly close together without the usual build-up of harmful tension in thigh muscles.

It is important not to seat children with their legs dangling; they should be given chairs of suitable height, or, failing that, some sort of platform to rest their feet on – at a pinch, you could make shift with telephone directories, provided they cover a large enough surface. The same advice applies to very short adults, and is often even more important than the height of work surfaces.

It will be seen that all the advice in this chapter depends on people sitting in a way that respects the integrity of the framework of the human body. **It is not possible to force anyone to sit sensibly, but it should be a matter for general concern that everyone should have the opportunity to do so.**

Wheelchairs, pushchairs

What are we to say, then, about some of the painfully awkward situations into which people are sometimes forced? Several times, when asked to help people in wheelchairs, I have been horrified to see sagging seats, backs that give no support, crushingly narrow armrests, nowhere to rest the head, and a stupid little bar that doesn't support the feet properly in any position, still less allow for any change of attitude. If to sit at a desk for hours can be felt sometimes as an intolerable constraint, what must it be like to spend one's waking hours in one of these contraptions? I know wheelchairs need to be light, for the sake of the people who have to push them; I know they must go through narrow doorways and that it must be possible to fold them into cars – but with modern materials and technology, surely it is not necessary to drive people still further into handicaps and discouragement. Some pushchairs are as bad; it is sad to see children hunched and helpless, too young to complain of this obstacle to healthy development.

Cars

My remarks about contact with the floor hold good when you are driving. The placing of pedals in cars can be extremely important. The stiffest legs I have yet seen in normally healthy people belonged to two young women of short-to-average build, as I am myself. Realizing that they both drove the same type of car, I sat in the driving seat and soon spotted the cause of the problem. The pedals were placed so high and so far forward that they could not be reached with the heels on the floor; this meant that all the time you were driving, you were constantly obliged to lift both legs and push. The car in question might have been all right for a man with long legs and large feet, but this was a miscalculation on the part of the makers, since for other reasons it was less likely to appeal to very tall people. You might not notice this snag until you had driven the car for a bit, so be warned.

Beds

It does now seem to be more or less generally understood that firm beds are healthier than soft ones. As I said when talking about chairs, it is not at all restful if you constantly have to adapt to the thing that is supposed to be supporting you. If for any reason you get landed with a really soggy mattress, it is better to put it on the floor than to wake up stiff and aching.

I sometimes get asked about the best position for sleeping – often by people who have taken my advice (in Chapter 28) a bit too much to heart. By all means lie down as described in that chapter, *before* you go to bed: you will be in a better state to start your night's rest. Then go to bed and forget about positions, for in any case a lot of movement goes on during healthy sleep. A few pointers are worth bearing in mind: if you sleep on your back or side, you will probably need two pillows, but if you turn on to your front during the night, push the pillows away. It is a good idea to remember, just before you go to sleep, that you don't really want to pull your head backwards – then, if you do so in your sleep, with practice you can programme yourself to come to the surface and change position. Don't be afraid to push your pillows around and get comfortable – you are not on parade! Avoid special pillows that 'support' your neck while letting your head drop away from it, whether backwards or sideways.

In this chapter we have looked at a few typical difficulties that can arise from what one might call basic equipment. In the next chapter we shall consider some problems relating to some of the sophisticated equipment more recently arrived on the scene.

CHAPTER 30

REPETITIVE STRAIN INJURY – ANOTHER APPROACH

'I was looking for a mouse.'
'A mouse?' she said, 'What do you mean?'
Well, of course, if she didn't know what a mouse was, there
was evidently a good deal of tedious spadework before us...
P.G. Wodehouse *Jeeves in the Offing*

Though my purpose in writing has been simply to present basic information that ought to be available to everyone, I cannot leave this discussion of mind and muscle without dealing specifically, however briefly, with the vexed question of Repetitive Strain Injury. At the time of writing, the term is used, mainly in the world of computers, to cover a set of conditions that cause a great deal of pain, undermining the health of many computer users. If you are one of those afflicted, you may have turned to this chapter before reading the rest of the book. That is very understandable, but I hope you will afterwards read the book from the beginning: my entire argument has a bearing on this painful problem, for which, believe me, *there are no quick fixes*.

Shortly after some computer operators had been awarded damages against their employers for what soon became known as RSI, a judge distinguished himself by saying that RSI didn't exist, and was duly ridiculed in the BBC's *Have I Got News For You*: '... when Judge So-and-so mistook himself for a medical expert' seemed to sum things up pretty neatly. Good grief, of course it exists. And some employers, while they try (not surprisingly) on the one hand to defend their financial interests, are at the same time sincerely searching for solutions. After all, nobody wants trouble if it can be avoided.

Sadly, the search so far has not been very fruitful. This is because it has usually been assumed that RSI is 'a new disease'. Specific conditions noted include tendonitis, frozen shoulder, bursitis, epicondylitis and carpal tunnel syndrome. Grouping these ailments under the one heading of 'Repetitive Strain Injury' provides an economical description, focusing attention accurately on a very real problem[1]. Most of my adult life has been spent in finding ways of avoiding this type of problem – first for myself, and later for others. So it is delightful to find it being given a name and being taken seriously. I only regret that the arguments about it have been so much beside the point.

The mistake has been to take the problem out of context, but it cannot have been easy to know just how to look at it. But when we take *Repetitive Strain Injury* to mean literally *injuries resulting from repeated strains on the organism*, we find evidence that such injuries existed in the mid-nineteenth century, when, for example, whole groups of mill-hands were found to be suffering from identical handicaps due to one particular re-peated action imposed by one particular job. This is well documented, but there are many ways in which repeated strain, or what I have called *unacceptable wear and tear* can be caused. Not all forms of wear and tear produce similar injuries (possibly Adam got lumbago and Eve suffered from spinner's thumb) but the symptoms listed above have long been familiar to musicians, as I have good reason to know. Perhaps because a typical day for me includes both types of work, I think a comparison between musicians and computer operators could yield useful pointers.

Musicians, like nineteenth-century factory workers, are not in a position to com-plain: even for good players, there are not too many jobs. If playing the violin for a living is excruciating, you don't say too much about it, or people will think you can't cope and will find another player who can. If you are very strongly motivated, you may start ques-tioning the technique you were taught as a youngster; if the pain gets too bad, you give up. Either way, it is a personal problem – or a personal failure, even a personal tragedy.

The situation changes when (as in the computer field) large numbers of decently paid people, similarly affected while using skills that are much in demand, feel com-pelled to complain. These people use machines that are constantly being improved: is it surprising if they look to technology to solve their own problems? But the difficulty is more complex than that; it is really about the *relationship* between man and the ma-chines he has created, between the equipment nature gave him and the equipment he has made for himself.

The very fact that it seems physically easy to press a light little key has quite a lot to do with the problem. I remember the first time I used an electric typewriter – the slight-est hesitation over how many m's in 'accommodation' and there you were with a couple of dozen of them. The lightness of the keys, though pleasant, does mean that you have to support your own hands and arms – the keyboard isn't going to help carry them for an instant, and additional gadgets don't help much.

The necessary support, which depends on a number of factors within the human body itself, has been extensively studied, though not, as it happens, in computer circles. So how is it possible to support the arms without strain? For example, how does a violin-ist keep both arms up hour after hour, while the fingers do complicated things? Some suffer tortures, while others are merely reasonably tired – what makes the difference? As explained elsewhere in this book, the performer who achieves economical support of the main structures of the body can undoubtedly command more freedom and agility in small precision movements.

The difficulties of working with a mouse are different from those presented by a key-board. Since the mouse will function even if you lean on it while collapsed in your chair, this may at first seem a reasonable way to work; perhaps you will find it restful – for a time. In the long term, it is you who will suffer, not the mouse – especially as it takes practice to acquire the co-ordination of hand and eye via the screen. It is highly inadvisable to practise it in ways that can only lay the foundations of future problems.

Let me issue a warning if you have any dealings with 'virtual reality'. This enormously interesting development has many exciting possibilities. Its use as a toy, however, can be dangerous: the human nervous system is designed to cope with *actual* reality. However serious your purpose, in working with the *virtual* variety, you will be well advised to organize your awareness so as to keep close track of what is happening to you in the real world. It may seem sometimes as though *only your brain* is working – but that brain, extended into all the nerves in your body, is inextricably entwined in muscle. You cannot avoid using your whole organism all the time, whatever your dominant preoccupation at any given moment.

Feedback is a key concept for the musician: the sounds we produce can tell us a lot about whether things are working properly. Another essential type of feedback comes from within, from the kinaesthetic sense, which tells us what we are doing muscularly. All this information can still be misused, for many factors tempt one into piling effort on effort in a misguided way. Alternatively, one can try to identify any *obstacles* to good performance, gradually learning to associate the results one hears with the means used to achieve them. The means include the instrument, one's own body, and one's thought processes. Using all these to the best advantage is what musicians call *technique*, of which the ear is supreme judge.

As a computer user, you do not have the advantage of the external feedback that musicians get from sound; but feedback from the kinaesthetic sense is there to let you know what is happening in your own body. You, too, need a *technique* for interpreting and using this type of feedback. You will need to become receptive to warning signals *before* they become pain, before they become strain, before they become injury. It will be necessary to acquire a habit of organizing your awareness so that those signals can reach consciousness soon enough to be useful. To heed them calls for a certain understanding of the workings of muscle; this understanding, and its practical application, is what this book is about.

Everyone can accept the idea that machines of all kinds must be used correctly or they will give trouble. The correct use of a machine is something that has to be learnt – you know about that; just as you know that the more versatile the machine, the more there is to learn about its various uses. The human organism can be adapted to many uses, but some of them really need to be studied. The analogy is exact. All the general guidelines given in this book are applicable.

There is no panacea – and no technology that could possibly protect you from the consequences of poor information about how mind and muscle interrelate in you personally. If any form of RSI is your problem, let me urge you to use your problem-solving skills in a way that includes in your field of awareness the question of *how you are using yourself*. By the way, don't make the mistake of supposing that the difficulty is peculiar to your particular kind of work. That is not only defeatist, it is also not true. It would be more accurate to say that your job is one of those most likely to bring you quickly and dramatically up against problems that are prevalent to some degree throughout our society – problems many of which are certainly associated with increasingly rapid technological change. That is why you need good information to enable you to exploit your adaptability as a human being.

The main text of this book explains the framework within which the astonishing human versatility can and must function. Here I would mention a few aspects that are particularly important for you to bear in mind. (You will find detailed explanations in the main text.)

1) *Head balance* (**Chapters 13–17**) inevitably influences our well-being in everything we do, therefore you must not be obliged to spend long periods craning your neck. So obviously your screen should be placed where you can see it conveniently, without pulling your head backwards. The same applies to any book or paper to which you refer frequently; there are various stands available which will hold documents at a convenient angle, so that you can also avoid stooping. Space for such necessities is as obvious a requirement as a decent light on your work. I am sure that you have given thought to such questions. It is still up to you to make good use of the space, the light, the aids, and – yourself. Ergonomics alone will never solve everything.

2) *Comfort* Anyone who works sitting down needs to be comfortably seated. But being 'comfortable' for work is not the same as lounging, so let me draw your attention to my explanation of balanced sitting (**Chapters 22–23**) as well as to what has been said about chairs. (**Chapter 29**)

3) The human body is superbly designed for versatility of movement; it is less fitted for *keeping still*, but that it can also manage. In fact, given the right conditions, it will treat keeping still as an extremely subtle form of movement. To give it that opportunity, from time to time spare a moment to think about movements we have discussed – even if you don't actually choose to do them just now, remember they are still available to you whenever you decide to use them. What you may be doing at a given moment may be fascinating, exacting, exasperating – but however busy you are, at least take a moment to look around you, to change the focus of your eyes, to pretend to yourself sometimes that you are just going to move, because this makes a physical difference. (**Chapter 9**) Of course, really move sometimes, too; any employer who misguidedly begrudges you the time to get up and move around a bit is not acting in his own best interests. Surely he wants you to be at your most efficient? How can you think properly if everything hurts?

4) Not only musicians, but people in your job, too, need to understand their *hands and arms*, and the supporting structure that is the shoulder girdle. (**Chapters 24–25–26**)

5) Prolonged *wrist flexion* is a dangerous habit. The fingers work best when the wrist is, as often as possible, slightly in extension. (**Chapter 26**)

6) Exaggerated *elbow flexion* is also dangerous. Use only just enough muscle power to give you the angle you want at your elbow – many people forget it is only a hand they are carrying, not the week's shopping.

7) *Habits* acquired in the course of one's work can be very strong. Avoid over-correcting. Try to identify things you do that may be harmful, and see whether you can do them less often. Notice if they occur at other times, when they are easier to relinquish. (**Chapter 32**)

8) *Prevention* is better than cure. Before difficulties become painful, give your body a chance to bounce back into shape. (**The quickest way is described in Chapter 28.**)

9) *Emotional stress* Deadlines, distractions, difficulties with colleagues, worries – whether personal, financial, or work-related – all or any of these can take their toll of one's health. Most people now recognize this – but knowing *that it happens* doesn't seem to solve much, in itself. But the better you understand *how* such problems may find expression in muscular behaviour, the better protected you will be. I have had this aspect in mind throughout writing this book. (**Chapters 9, 10, 33 may help you to see the point of some of the more detailed information and advice given in other chapters.**)

10) *Boredom* Sometimes, though one may not care to admit it, pressures of work may be compounded by boredom. (I know all about that: I once played the same musical comedy for two years and a half!) *Bored stiff, bored to tears, bored to extinction* – the colloquialisms hardly exaggerate the damaging effects of boredom. Its only saving feature is that it does give you the opportunity of noticing how you are using yourself; and that, when approached constructively, is highly interesting.

---

1. Amazingly, some people are still unwilling to recognize *use* as a factor. I do not suggest that repetitive strain is the only possible cause of the conditions mentioned. (A kitten's claw once punctured the tip of my elbow, which rapidly became very inflamed and swollen; the diagnosis was *acute bursitis*.) However, this discussion – like so many – must turn ultimately on probabilities, experience and common sense.

CHAPTER 31

EXERCISE AND EXERCISES

Consider the auk;
Becoming extinct because he forgot how to fly and could only walk.
Consider man, who may well become extinct
Because he forgot how to walk and learned to fly before he thinked.

Ogden Nash *A caution to everybody*

... misuse has got to be eliminated before it makes sense to try and
build something up... Progress in athletic performance comes through
increasing the demand on yourself while ensuring the full, intelligent,
conscious response to the demand that the direction, co-ordination and
balance are meanwhile correctly maintained.

Walter Carrington *Thinking Aloud*

Many people in our society, bored with working in an increasingly artificial, mechanized environment, place a high value on leisure activities of all kinds. Sooner or later they become aware that it is some time since they did anything that really called for the expenditure of physical energy. They notice feeling better after a holiday or a day spent walking or cycling in the country – they may even feel rather pleased with themselves after catching a bus they had to run for, or moving the furniture around, or doing a bit of gardening. But sometimes these things make them breathless, or they pull a muscle, or end up with backache. And so come the questions. *Am I getting out of condition? Ought I to take more exercise? What kind of exercise would be good for me?* These are good questions, emanating from a sound instinct.

However, these questions frequently take the form of suggesting forms of exercise that would be unwise in the circumstances – and it can be quite hard to give sensible advice without sounding discouraging. The people concerned sometimes have such obvious faults in their management of themselves that to ask more of the 'framework' in its present state would exaggerate the faults to danger point. (If your car is in need of service, you might risk it as far as the local shops, but would you dare rely on it to take you on holiday in the Alps?) Yet I do agree that we all need to move. Perhaps it is our ideas about exercise that need to be revised.

Exercise for what? To get fit, of course. So – what is 'fit'? I would define it as being able to do what you need to do, and what you want to do, while feeling up to what you expect of yourself – and this of course varies considerably from one person to another.

What is usually called 'fitness' seems to have two main aspects. One, *cardiovascular* fitness, has to do with the heart and the blood vessels: how much, and how energetically, can I move before I get out of breath, before I get a stitch, before my heart races and my limbs feel weak and nothing seems to work any more? This type of fitness is cultivated by regular demands on the system. In recent years, it has often been pointed out that in a largely sedentary society, people who take regular exercise have a better life expectancy. I am not going to start disputing that: all those insurance companies can't have got their sums wrong – their money is at stake, for goodness' sake!

The other kind of fitness, generally thought of as *muscular*, concerns the skeletal muscles. Of course the two kinds of fitness are related, but the distinction should not be ignored. It is possible to train yourself into a fair standard of cardiovascular fitness (at any rate, for a time) while simultaneously damaging your framework, of which the system of skeletal muscles forms an important part. People who do this tend not to pay serious attention to questions of *muscular* fitness until they encounter problems, which are then regarded as 'injuries' and therefore considered to be a medical matter. But if A is injured while doing something that B does with impunity, the question that *should* arise is, was it really an accident, or was A not 'fit' to do it? When the crunch comes, even A's cardiovascular fitness probably suffers, too, because defects in the framework, (including its muscular components) force him or her to stop activities that the organism as a whole has got used to. Quite often, A decides either a) that he wasn't fit enough in the first place, and should do more warming-up exercises in future, or b) that it was just bad luck – so when the effects of injury recede after a period of rest, he will work hard to get 'fit' again. Does he think much about the right way to do a particular exercise, or whether it will suit him personally?

Yet, as we have seen, the *how* is at least as important as the *what*. There are many forms of exercise, enjoyable and healthy for people who make good use of the framework, that I would hesitate to recommend to people with certain types of difficulty. The essential question is: *on what basis is the system habitually being used?* If misuse is habitual, weightlifting, for example, will exaggerate the misuse; in this case, quite seriously, it would be better exercise to pick up a pin with due regard to the fundamentals of good co-ordination. (Chapters 10–26 show just how many considerations can affect such a simple action!) *All day long, every little thing you do is either good or bad exercise, according to how you do it.*

This being so, it stands to reason that any specific exercise is only good or harmful in relation to the condition of the person practising it. Here is a rather striking example. Some time before I knew him, a young athlete had been forced to give up running, because of a knee injury. After an operation, followed by physiotherapy, he had become a keen and good swimmer. He consulted me about a pain in the shoulder, which was affecting one of his strokes. In passing, he mentioned that he was continuing to do the postoperative exercise he had been given to strengthen the quadriceps of the injured leg. I asked him to demonstrate the exercise, and was startled to observe enough misuse of the head/neck/shoulder area to account for the shoulder problem. My next task might have been to help him to do the leg exercise without harming the shoulder – but first I used standard tests to determine whether this particular exercise was still necessary. The man was amazed and amused to find that the quadriceps of his 'weak' leg had now become *slightly too strong* and that he had been diligently damaging his shoulder to no purpose at all – and to the detriment of his new sport.

The above is an example of the kind of thing that can very easily happen if one does any exercise without taking into account what is happening to the rest of the framework. This case, of a problem arising out of an exercise begun in the first instance under medical advice, shows why specific exercises of any kind, however necessary, should only be used with due attention to their total effect. How much more is this true when people with insufficient information at their disposal decide on an exercise they think will be good for them! I am thinking of all those abdominal exercises that are supposed to firm up the tummy, but end by restricting rib movement; of toe-touching (if you can do it, you don't need to make an exercise of it; if you can't, watch out – you could damage your spine by insisting); of head-rolling exercises (done with the idea of 'freeing the neck') which only confuse the reflexes that balance the head (see Chapter 16); of breathing exercises (see Chapters 11 and 12); of shoulder exercises that distort the shoulder girdle; of arm exercises that weaken the back instead of contributing to its strength, and so on. Some people practise sit-ups, in the hope of curbing a bulging abdomen: they risk a) shortening hip flexors that are already too short, b) disturbing the balance between the front and back of the trunk, with consequent danger to the spine[1] and c) defeating their own purpose by reducing the space available for the tidy stowing of abdominal contents.

People do so many of these things that ultimately detract from their fitness. They do them with the best of intentions – and often feel good for a while, but that feeling tends not to last long if the well-being of the whole has not been adequately considered. No, for most people it is better to do things for fun, as I have said before, and never mind all this working hard to 'do yourself good'. We use ourselves better when having fun.

That being said, I have a great deal of sympathy for athletes who make courageous efforts to get back into form after injury – they work themselves so hard, often in the teeth of considerable pain. Sometimes on television one sees well-known athletes struggling in a way that fills me with a mixture of respect, compassion and frustration. Here, perhaps, is someone who before injury was superbly co-ordinated – not only for a particular sport but in daily life – which partly explains the original success. Alas, what we have called 'good use of the framework' was at first so natural to the person concerned that its essence went unrecognized, even by the owner. Hence, the fundamental co-ordination, once compromised by adaptations to an injury, is difficult to regain. I sincerely hope that what I have written may start such people directing their efforts along different lines. In sport, as in many other fields of endeavour, much serious work has been done to improve *specific techniques*. Again as in other fields, more reference could fruitfully be made to the fundamental organization of the human frame necessary for *any* healthy activity – such organization could usefully be regarded as a *pre-technique*.

Awareness of this need for a pre-technique is what I would urge on anyone starting any kind of 'get fit' programme, at any level. If you have stayed with me so far, you know something about which functions need to be available, you know about not impeding reflex action. You know, too, that any kind of strained effort shows up in the relationship of head to neck – that highly important indicator – and that this is a matter of personal understanding and personal responsibility. I should like to give just a few examples of how this knowledge can be applied in practice.

Walking and running are of course two of the most readily available forms of exercise. Until very recent times, they were obvious and necessary ways of getting from place to place. Walking was an important part of my wartime childhood, though the long walk to and from school was not very enjoyable, because of a heavy satchel to carry. On the other hand, it was highly agreeable to step out empty-handed to go and play with a friend a couple of miles away. I wonder how many people nowadays know the pleasure of getting into your stride, with the natural swing of your arms to help you along. I can recommend it, particularly in fields or park or woods, with clean air and plenty to look at – but even in town, in quieter streets, it is possible to get into a rhythm. (I know a man with two offices, who walks empty-handed from one to the other: having first faxed the papers he needs, he can dispense with a brief-case and enjoy the walk.)

You see, our arms do not cease to be forelegs, just because we no longer go on all fours.[2] The cross-pattern relationship between arms and legs, present from the moment we started to crawl (creep, in American) still has a good deal of importance (**Chapter 20**). For one thing it helps our balance; for another, the arm movement acts on the length of stride; thirdly, by creating a gentle and natural diagonal stretch, it continues the good work that crawling did for our backs when we were little. Here are some experiments, to be done out of doors for preference. You will, of course, gain more from them if you bear in mind the importance of a freely-balancing head.

❑ *Experiment 1*

With arms folded behind your back, run fairly quickly, for about 25 metres. Most people are astonished to find how much, and how spontaneously, their shoulders move, making up for the fact that the arms are no longer free to compensate for first one leg, then the other being in front.

❑ *Experiment 2*

(to be done at moderate speed, on a fairly steep slope)
a) Walk uphill with your arms rigidly at your sides.
b) Walk uphill with your arms hanging freely, neither willing a swing, nor preventing it if it happens.
c) Walk uphill, definitely swinging your arms in very big movements. What was the effect on your stride? Vary the speed of arm-swinging. What happened?
d) Try a) b) and c) in a run, if you feel like it.
e) Run downhill. What happened to your arms? Can they regulate speed or length of stride? Can they have a braking effect?

You could investigate these questions as you walk. You could also think about Experiment 3 in Chapter 18, extending it to include observations of the effect of different types of terrain. Remember, too, that in learning from babies (**Chapter 20**) we noticed that the flexion/extension movements of hip and knee are closely related to rotation of the thigh-bone in the hip-joint. Above all, remember the freedom of the head. With all this to think about, and your surroundings to look at, I don't think walking will be boring for you, even if some people find it so.

If you want to get pleasure from *running*, I suggest that the first positive step is to find a good natural rhythm for walking. When you start to enjoy walking fairly fast, one day when you are having a good time and feeling a bit exuberant, let your walk spill over into running. It isn't cheating to run downhill! Run while you want to, not more, but – and this is very important – **don't stop abruptly**. If you are tired or out of breath, on no account go 'oof!' and collapse into a slump; you should take the pressure off yourself *gradually*, by walking briskly for a bit, then perhaps more gently. Experienced athletes know about this, of course, but people new to the exercise idea may not be aware that it is dangerous to ignore this rule, particularly if you are not in excellent condition. If you run when you feel like it, and change to a brisk walk before you are tired of running, you may well find that you can enjoy more of it as your condition improves. Alternate walking and running as you please, but always start and finish by walking.

As you can see, walking and running are naturally related, and many of the same things apply to both. I have never been fond of the term 'jogging', which seems to imply heaviness, and up-and-down rather than forward movement. *(Jog – run at a slow pace, esp. as physical exercise; proceed laboriously, trudge; move up and down with an unsteady motion, O.E.D.)* All really good movement has an element of lightness, a springy quality throughout the organism. Many of us have known something of this quality at some time in our lives; I think the aim of rightly directed exercise of any kind should be to re-discover it.

These remarks about running owe a lot to my long association with another Alexander teacher, the late Paul Collins, whose story is worth repeating here. Paul was three times Canadian marathon champion and represented Canada in the 1952 Olympics, but a severe knee injury then forced him out of international competition. Paul really loved running, so he tried every available treatment, but all his attempts to run again ended in frustration until the late 1960's, when he saw that he must challenge his basic assumptions about running and movement generally. I well remember the day when, dissatisfied with his speed on a training run, he decided, rather than trying to run faster, to pay more attention to how he was using his whole framework – and discovered presently that he was running faster without particularly meaning to. Encouraged, he persisted in this approach and eventually became attracted by the challenge of ultra-long distances. Thirty years after the original injury, during a six-day race, I saw him break ten world records for his veteran group. At the post-race medical check, the doctor remarked that Paul was the only athlete in the race who had not needed medical attention at some time during that week. It may seem a rather extreme way of proving that use affects functioning, but he made his point!

Swimming For those who enjoy it (as I do, very much) swimming is generally recognized to be an excellent exercise for the whole body. The change in the effect of gravity offers possibilities that we don't have on land, while the very fact of being in a different element imposes certain restrictions on any tendency to sudden, jerky movements. For these reasons, certain convalescents can begin to make movements in the water that are impossible for them in our usual environment. Why then is it that many people say they like the water but tend to get a 'stiff neck' after swimming? Clearly, it is because they have never questioned their belief that they need to '*lift the head out of the water* in order to breathe in'. In my terms, this means *to pull the head backwards* – which does not suit the human organism any better in water than out of it; indeed, to a large extent, it im-pedes movement and makes breathing itself more difficult! This is where more up-to-date swimming techniques can help basic co-ordination (though, oddly enough, some swimmers who know all about them do not seem aware of all the possibilities they offer).

As a child, I was told that in breast-stroke the arm movement was *forward, then side-ways*. (Even today, this is sometimes taught.) If you do that, I agree that you will have to pull your head backwards when you need air (or else remain vertical in the water, which won't get you far!) As serious swimmers know, the proper way to do this stroke is: after the forward movement of the arms, there is an important *downward* element in bringing the hands back to the breast. In the thirty years or so since I first learnt this, the precise details of the stroke have varied with further discoveries in aquadynamics, but the point I want to make is this: *as a result of the downward arm movement, your head clears the water automatically, without any need to pull it backwards for breathing in.* Try it: it is more comfortable, the limb movements become stronger – and you will get along better without the braking effect caused by the backward movement of the head. Of course, during the 'arms forward' part of the stroke, you must not mind getting your face wet – if you breathe out when it is in the water, that is not really a problem.

Nevertheless, many people do have a strong habit of pulling the head backwards when swimming; usually, the habit was formed when, as children, they were a bit scared of the whole thing. If you like swimming, and would like to tackle this habit, I think you will be interested in Chapters 32 and 33, which deal respectively with obstacles due to habits and fears.

As I have implied elsewhere, we all have habits whose reason for existing we may well have forgotten. If some of them get in our way, what are we to do? We have touched on this before; in Chapter 32, we go further into the question.

---

1. F.P. Kendall and E.K. McCreary, *Muscles – Testing and Function*, Baltimore, Williams and Wilkins, 3rd edition, 1983, p. 207, 'Sit-up Exercises: Indications and Contraindications':
    '... The possibility exists that the knee-bent sit-up, in which the hip flexors shorten to a greater extent than with the legs extended, may be even more conducive to developing shortness in the muscles and increasing the lordosis ... The people most in danger of being adversely affected ... are children and youths ... Those adults who have low back pain that is associated with excessive low back flexibility also may be affected adversely by this ... *some subjects show excessive flexion in sitting or forward bending, but a lordosis in standing.*' (My italics) 'It is unfortunate that the ability to do a certain number of sit-ups, re-gardless of how they are performed, is used as a measure of physical fitness.'
    Personally, I find it astonishing that such warnings, from such a respected source, still go largely un-heeded.
2. This was pointed out by Percy Cerutty, coach of world-class athletes.

Chapter 32

HABIT

... I am swallowed up by things customary ... so much
does the burden of custom count for.

St. Augustine *Confessions*

To improve as much as I have done this year, you first
have to accept the possibility of playing a lot worse.

Virginia Wade (on winning the Wimbledon title)

Habit is not inherited. It is not 'reflex action'.

Sir Charles Sherrington *Man on his Nature*

Anyone who experiments with movement of any kind, for whatever reason, certainly encounters, sooner or later, a whole network (often amounting to a 'net to trap the unwary') constructed of his or her own habits. We are all familiar with the distinction between 'good' and 'bad' habits, but to categorize them in this way is only part of the story. Potential helps and hindrances can exist in a single habit. Habits are certainly useful for saving time, enabling us to carry out learnt sequences without constantly reconsidering basic procedures; enabling us, also, to construct new skills on the basis of past achievement. But even 'good' habits can be a nuisance at moments when they are inappropriate. (I remember with shame how once, in the middle of a prolonged drought, on a farm miles from anywhere and dependent on its own well, I only *just* managed to stop myself from flushing the lavatory, although it had been carefully explained that frequent flushing could lead to the calamity of an empty well.)

Sometimes, too, good habits have been acquired in a job lot of extraneous material. As a child, 'helping' in the kitchen, it was by watching my mother that I learnt how to beat eggs with a fork. Along with the rapid forearm movement, I copied what she did with her shoulders – and soon began to feel cramped and tired. How could I know, young as I was, that the tension I had copied was merely an expression of my mother's anxiety to hurry on to the next task, that it contributed nothing to the speed or effectiveness of the egg-beating? Whipping up the *whites* of eggs was done with a knife on a large plate, but since this skill, even more fascinating, was demonstrated by my grandmother, a dignified old lady who operated at her own speed, it never involved me in muscular problems, then or later. As an adult, I have been able to analyse the difference, and have become passionately interested in disentangling skills from the snares surrounding them.

The particular little challenge I have just described was rather fun to tackle, but people often find that the habits they want to change seem really compulsive, as though a particular way of doing something were some kind of drug. Indeed, there is a certain similarity between the problem of the smoker who can't give up, and that of, shall we say, the sufferer from back pain who, aware that a false move may bring disaster, nevertheless feels compelled to move in the habitual way. 'The reflex is so strong' they say – for someone in this quandary will often use the words 'reflex' and 'habit' as though they were synonymous, which is far from being the case. Turning to the dictionary again, we find the following:

1) **Reflex** – an action independent of the will, as an automatic response to the stimulation of a nerve (e.g. a sneeze).
2) **Habit** – a settled disposition or tendency to act in a certain way, esp. one acquired by frequent repetition of the same act; a practice that is hard to give up; a mental constitution or attitude.

Reflexes are reactions implanted by nature; they help and protect us. Habits are quasi-automatic reactions in which we have drilled ourselves, either on purpose or inadvertently. The relationship between the two is complex and the degree of control we have over either is variable, but I am sure it is important to distinguish between them, and to know the extent of the domain in which we have some freedom of choice.

In certain circumstances, *pace* the dictionary, one can override a reflex by a conscious decision. This may be likened to what one does when, in dealing with machinery, one interrupts the action of an automatic device, so as to take manual control. Thus, though coughing and sneezing are reflex actions designed by nature to rid the body of unwanted matter, the operation of the reflex can sometimes be delayed or suppressed out of consideration for others. Breathing itself can be interrupted temporarily, if it is necessary to pass through a bad smell. Furthermore, while it is of course natural to withdraw from a painful contact (which is why you may drop a plate that is burning you) the conscious wish to avoid smashing the plate and spilling your food may enable you to override the natural reaction for long enough to reach the table. In infants, for whom falling represents such danger, the dominant *grasping reflex* (Chapter 33) may *prevent* the release of a pain-causing object, but as adults, we do acquire a certain amount of practical experience relating to reflex mechanisms. We know (usually non-verbally) something about their usefulness and its limitations. With a little more understanding, it is possible to enlarge this experiential knowledge, to know better when it is safe to override a reflex, and when the wisest course is to get out of the way and let the reflex operate.

Oddly enough, we are often more apt to submit to our habits than to our reflexes. And though you may not *intend* to override reflex functioning, some habits do have that effect, with unfortunate results. I explained (in Chapter 14) that the unintentional pulling backwards of the head, at its joint with the atlas, impedes the head's all-important reflex balancing act. Sad to say, this habit is so prevalent (for reasons see Chapter 33) and has such far-reaching effects, that it must be confronted whenever any serious attempt at change is decided upon.

If you want to experiment with unfamiliar ways of doing anything, I would recommend the following plan.

1) Accept that it is of the very nature of an experiment that success is not necessarily implied – the whole idea is to find out what happens if you approach things differently.

2) Give yourself adequate time, for no true experiment can be made (or evaluated) by someone who is trying to rush.

3) Remember that pulling the head backwards would be *the* fundamental mistake, upsetting the balance not only of the head itself but of the whole framework within and around which the chosen action will occur. This, therefore, had better be your primary consideration. (**Chapter 17**)

4) Continue to bear this in mind while being as clear as possible about any secondary mistakes you have specifically decided to avoid. (If you have worked through the experiments in this book so far, you will have found some of them pretty obvious and others more tricky. So by now you probably have a fair idea which mistakes concerning the framework are most likely to lie in wait for you personally.)

5) While you consider the task ahead, remember that points 3) and 4) continue to be relevant.

6) Then, still avoiding the most likely pitfalls, particularly with regard to the head – have a go! Don't at this point enter into a lot of detail about precisely *how* the action is to be carried out: by avoiding the worst pitfalls you will anyway have created a different framework for the movements you are going to make. In these changed circumstances, the movements themselves may differ substantially from your expectations. After all, you are *experimenting*.

7) Afterwards, you can criticize the result if you like, but *don't at this stage try to monitor a movement while doing it*, or you will risk slowing it down to an unnatural degree, which is always harder.

Let me expand this a little. It is clear, when you come to think about it, that for every movement there is a speed that is the most natural and therefore the easiest. This speed is largely related to your physical proportions. A little child takes smaller, quicker steps than a tall man; to imitate each other would be tiring for both, if not impossible. It would be very hard work to swing your arms as rapidly as you drum on the table with your fingers. To slow down the drumming of your fingers to a comfortable speed for arm-swinging would stiffen you, destroying the smooth rhythm of the movement. Large movements are slow; small movements are quick, for the speed of a movement depends very much on the size and weight of the moving part, as well as on fluctuations in your energy and in the state of your general co-ordination. Granted that it may be necessary, for all sorts of reasons, to modify the speed of a movement, it is always advisable to start by discovering what seems *a natural speed for you, today* – so that you have a standard of ease, from which you depart as little as is consistent with what you want to accomplish.

I expect it is in doing something challenging, something you care about, that you are likely to want to introduce improvements – a sport, perhaps, or playing a musical instrument, or overcoming a handicap of some kind. This provides excellent motivation, but it can be discouraging to go headlong into trying to improve actions that you already know to be problematic. This is because improvement means change, and change means being able to set aside the habitual; and that – until the experimental sorting process has progressed further – can mean a temporary loss of *useful* elements of the habitual pattern, along with those you would be happy to discard. To face this apparent loss, in the context of something that is important to you, you need a fair amount of confidence in yourself *and in the process*. This being so, there is a lot to be said for practising your experimental skills on things you already do easily, things you take for granted, things that are not emotionally charged: they will provide more encouraging material for the application of the principles described here. And if a given experiment happens to prove non-productive, it is easier to be casual about it.

You know yourself and your own life, so the best ideas for experimental material will be the ones you think up yourself – but, to start you off, here are a few suggestions.

❏ *Experiment 1*

Having given yourself time to let your head balance itself freely, try lifting a hand to brush your hair back, without disturbing your head. Did the hand go all the way, or did your head come halfway to meet it? Obviously, there is no absolute right or wrong about this, but it is interesting to see how much choice you have (or haven't) in making such a trivial gesture. Just *because* it is trivial, you can have fun experimenting – fun that you might deny yourself if you were dealing with something that mattered.

❏ *Experiment 2*

Using the same approach as above, lift a glass to your lips. If you are sitting, put the glass back on the table by opening your elbow, rather than by bending forward. If you are standing when you put down the glass, think first about the head, then see if your legs, rather than your waist, will fold a little. It may feel odd but never mind – it doesn't look it.

It is a good idea to invent for yourself small challenges of this kind, to play with in the course of the day's routine. Try to think up a new one each day, chosen from the repertoire of things for which you have formed habits, things that normally don't demand any attention. The most useful aspect of the game is the tiny pause that gives you time to think about your head. (Chapters 13–17) Probably you won't always *take* the opportunity to do so, but at least the chance will be there. In this way, bit by bit, you build up experience that will stand you in good stead when you seriously want to change the way you do something.

Finally, I should like to propose an experiment that is more difficult, because it concerns something we all practised with some care at a time when our co-ordination was not fully equal to it, that is: ***writing***. A cramped use of the hand is often seen in children – and in adults, too (fig. 55). Things that have been deliberately practised are often particularly resistant to change, so a method for dealing with this type of problem may prove useful to you.

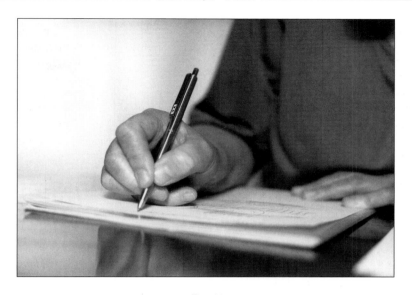

— Fig. 55 —
A cramped use of the hand

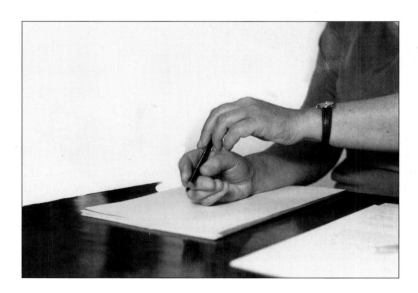

— Fig. 56 —
Passive hand receiving a pencil

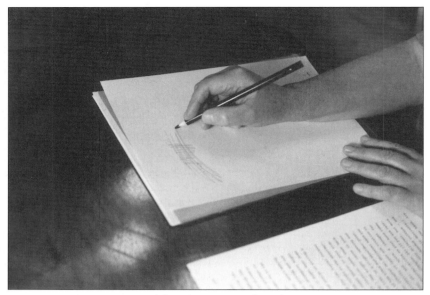

a) lateral movements from the wrist

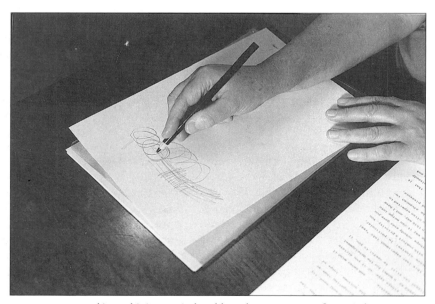

b) combining vertical and lateral movements to form circles

_ *Fig. 57* _
Learning to scribble

224

❏ *Experiment 3*

NB Use a *pencil* when you first do this experiment. Leave until later any similar experimenting with pens, ball-points, etc.

1. Sitting comfortably at a desk or table, place a sheet of paper in front of you, not centrally but nearer to the hand you write with.
2. Pause for a moment's thought about your head. Still thinking about your head, move the writing hand first into Neutral Readiness (**Chapter 26**) then open your elbow so that your hand (still in NR) rests lightly on the paper.
3. Pause again. Still thinking about your head and its freedom, use your other hand to pass a pencil to your writing hand, which remains passively receptive while the pencil is placed in it (fig. 56). If the pencil does not feel right in your hand ... pause again, as this is a crucial moment. (So please, don't start wondering if you could ever write like this!)
4. Instead, release your head from anything that might be pulling it down towards your hand, and adjust the pencil, if necessary, with your other hand, so that it touches the pads (not the very tips) of index and thumb, and rests on the side of the second finger, near the nail.
5. Still giving your head permission to balance freely, pronate the writing forearm slightly. This should bring the point of the pencil into some kind of contact with the paper, but don't worry if it doesn't: just use the other hand to make adjustments to the pencil, as before.
6. Never forgetting your head, play about with dots, dashes and exclamation marks. What type or types of tiny movement get the pencil off the page again, and in what circumstances? (Wrist extension? Forearm supination? The curve implicit in every flexion or extension of the fingers and thumb?)
7. Still giving some thought to the head, straighten the thumb and first two fingers, so as to make a slight *upward* mark on the paper. The mark will possibly be faint, but please make it as large as the straightening of the fingers and thumb will allow. Your contact with the pencil should be just enough to prevent it slipping away, no more. The thumb is the positive mover; the fingers, passive, let themselves be guided by it.
8. Still present in your head, casually allow your fingers and thumb to flex a little. You will probably find that all it takes to bring them back – enough to make a small downward mark on the paper – is: not to continue positively straightening them.
9. Continuing to refer to your head, you can start repeating the flexion/extension movements of steps 7 and 8, *still making the up-stroke the positive movement*. The result is a gentle scribble that could be said to correspond vaguely to vertical strokes in writing. On no account start pressing the index finger on to the pencil – you should just barely feel the contact.
10. Still according dominance to the head's easy poise, start making lateral movements from the wrist (fig. 57a). (If you were writing and not just scribbling, the result of these lateral movements might have something to do with crossing 't's, or it might bear some relation to travelling along the page in the course of writing a word.)

11. If you are right-handed, you will find you can travel further still by letting the head of the *humerus* rotate in the shoulder-joint in such a way that your elbow comes nearer to your side. (Left-handers will find that this rotation takes them back towards the beginning of the line.) The slight curve in your scribble can be corrected, if you like, by a slight opening and closing (extension and flexion) of the elbow and shoulder joint, so keep these options open, too. (**Chapter 26**) Don't lean on your hand. Whichever hand you write with, do check the availability of upper arm rotation in the shoulder joint (**Chapter 25**) and spare a thought for maintaining the width of the shoulder girdle as your hand comes nearer to the centre of your body. (**Chapter 24**) (If you are left-handed, writing movements will be not only different, but more difficult – like most things in a right-handed culture – and attention to these precautions is particularly desirable.)

12. With head still very easy and far away from the hand, try different ways of combining vertical and lateral scribbles (9 and 10 above) into rough clockwise and anticlockwise circles. Vary their size and don't bother if they encroach on each other.

13. Then travel a bit, adding some half-circles, higher or lower. (Some of this might begin to look a bit like eeeeeeee, aaaaaaaa, or ooooooooo in joined-up writing.)

14. Elongate the circles into loops, so that they become rather like llllllll joined-up.

15. Still within the same framework of poised head and easy hand, try some figure-of-eight movements, gradually elongating them so that the tops become loops of 'h's and the bottoms, loops of 'g's.

And so on, as easily and playfully as possible – and never mind if you prefer italic script, or if you always type, or if you dictate everything to your secretary. Viewed as a model for the development of existing skills, this experiment can still be useful to you, if faithfully carried out.

Don't be in a hurry to develop this last experiment into 'real writing': the emerging ease can prove elusive! In particular, reducing the size should be done gently, with comfort a priority. You have years of experience of writing, but perhaps nobody ever gave you time to learn enough about *scribbling* and the way it can merge into comfortable writing. Most of us have suffered in this way, and I have always thought it a great pity that children are so often expected to write properly before they have even acquired the advanced co-ordination needed for handling a pencil with ease and pleasure.

The principal value of Experiment 3 is that it demonstrates a plan for reconsidering skills that are already established, a *modus operandi* for digging up long-buried habits and taking another look at them. The procedure may seem finicky in the first instance, but subsequent application involves less loss of time than might be supposed. *The reason I have insisted on the freedom of the head as the preparation for each and every experimental step is that the head/neck area is where any contradictions in your co-ordination will announce their presence. Conversely, when you succeed in calming this area, reassuring ripples from the 'good example' tend to spread to the rest of your system.* It is precisely this that Professor John Dewey had in mind, when, in *Human Nature and Conduct*, he drew the conclusion:

Until one takes intermediate acts seriously enough to treat them as ends, one wastes one's time in any effort at change of habits. Of the intermediate acts, the most important is the *next* one. The first or earliest means is the most important *end* to discover.[1]

Essentially, this is work you do yourself, but if initially you feel that individual advice from a teacher would be helpful, I hope you won't be shocked or astonished – you aren't the only one! Admittedly, F.M. Alexander did this sort of thing – and much more – when working to solve his voice problem, and he did it alone. But many ordinary mortals, and some extraordinary ones, too (**see Chapter 34**) find they can use some expert help, if only to save time. Alone or with a teacher, *you* know which are the habits you would particularly like to reconsider. The procedure described above is a tried and tested way of going about it.

There is one main obstacle to successful change. There is a sense, implied in Virginia Wade's remark quoted above, in which 'the good is the enemy of the best'. It is neatly illustrated by a true story. I was once asked to take a look at a little girl of four, who had been learning the violin for just one month. She liked it and was getting along quite well, despite (like me at the same age) holding both violin and bow in a very awkward way that would certainly have to be unlearnt at some stage – and the sooner, the easier. In fact, it wasn't at all difficult to get her holding them absolutely perfectly, whereupon she cried, 'But Mummy, like this I can't play my little tunes any more!' I contrast this with a pleasant memory of working with a well-known cellist who had asked me to comment on his way of using himself while playing. I did not want to rush in where angels fear to tread (after all, he was the cellist, not me) nor did I want to risk saying anything that might disturb his performance that evening. However, he said he had done so much experimenting that he was confident of being able to try any suggestions of mine, and to use them or not, as he chose. His attitude is rare: most of us, like that child, spontaneously cling to what we know, to what we can do already, to our familiar habits, as though something precious were at risk. In various ways, the perception of *change as danger* seems almost universal. This is why in Chapter 33 we shall be considering the relationship between muscles and fear.

---

1. J. Dewey, *Human Nature and Conduct (an introduction to social psychology)* New York, Holt, 1922.

MUSCLES AND FEAR

> ... unable to think for fear, and ready to run anywhere to
> elude the awful creature... she rushed straight out of the
> gate and up the mountain. It was foolish indeed ... as if
> she had been seeking a fit spot for the goblin-creature to
> eat her in at his leisure; but that is the way fear serves us: it
> always sides with the thing we are afraid of.
>
> George MacDonald *The Princess and the Goblin*

When people begin to accept the extent to which mistakes have been made in our use of ourselves, they often ask how it is possible that such widespread confusion could arise. To understand what goes wrong, I think we need to look at some of the earliest reactions of babyhood and how they influence adult life.

One of the great dangers to a young baby is that it may fall or be dropped on its head. If our evolutionary ancestors were tree-dwellers, this danger must have been even more significant. Be that as it may, nature has provided the infant with a reflex response to the sensation of falling.[1] The arms are first flung wide, then brought near the body again.[2] The tiny hands will close in their surprisingly strong reflex grip on anything they happen to touch – perhaps they will find something useful to clutch. If so, the grip will tighten, involving a strong enough flexion of the whole upper limb to support the weight of the body.[3]

Suppose there is nothing to hold on to – what then? In particular, what of the head, proportionately heavier than an adult's? Surely it will crash first to the ground? Testing these reflexes artificially must be extremely difficult. (If a baby really falls, who on earth bothers with anything but trying to save it? A natural reluctance to subject babies to dangerous experiments may explain the dearth of detail in the available descriptions.) There seems, however, to be general agreement on certain points. One is that from the outset, *the head has been thrown backwards*, and the back arched. (*See note 2.*) One might think that this implies a backward fall on to the head – so what is the advantage? – except that in the initial phase, while the arms are seeking safety, we may suppose that the extension (arching) of the back is preparing a stronger flexing (forward bending) than would otherwise have been possible; and that this will give the head some chance of being protected in a backward fall by the rounded mass of the body. The abduction of the arms (in phase one) presumably invites an extra intake of breath, which will partly absorb the shock of a fall, should one occur. Not good, but better than nothing. This reflex reaction – part of our evolutionary inheritance – seems to be Nature's emergency solution to the threat which falling poses to the tiny baby.[4] (It has been suggested that tree-dwelling primates who did not react in this way were gradually eliminated in the course of evolution.)

Sudden changes of position in space are registered by a mechanism in the inner ear – so it is not surprising to find that, early in life, a sudden loud noise will produce a similar reaction. Thus our earliest fears appear related in a way that reinforces the reaction. Falling remains an emotionally loaded experience: people have nightmares about falling from a height; often someone who has got hurt by missing a step will tell you about it in a way that shows how disturbing it was. (I remember that once, replying to a friendly 'how was your day?' I mentioned having tripped on a cobble. I didn't bother to say that I had also that day burnt my tongue really badly – the fall, not particularly painful, seemed uppermost in my mind.)

It seems that the infant response to falling, so necessary for our protection when we were tiny, left such an impression on us that other fears became hooked up to it by association – and later in life a part of us often tries to respond in the same way, however inappropriately.[5,6] Adult reactions to fear or anxiety have this much in common with infant reactions to the sensation of falling: *a backward tilt of the head is associated with generalized flexor action in trunk and limbs*. These classic reactions, be they marked or subtle, have been part of the nitty-gritty of my working life for the past thirty years. I have had to recognize and deal with them in myself; I have had to suggest to others, directly or indirectly, some practical ways of coping with them. Between infant and adult, there are obvious differences as to how these manifestations are brought about. But I am convinced that the similarities have practical significance.

In very frightening situations people can be 'doubled up with fear', their 'legs give way under them' – which seems reminiscent of the flexion of the second phase of the infant reaction to falling. This is only the tip of the iceberg – and perhaps not the worst of it, because an adult who has experienced such extreme fear usually knows it and is conscious of the need to recover. More insidious – and devastatingly common – are the problems arising from a modified version of the reaction. Examples are all around us, so familiar that we hardly notice the signs in ourselves or in others. Sudden loud noises, traffic emergencies, pain, shyness, stage fright, hidden anger combined with fear at our own aggressive tendencies... many and frequent are the stimuli that produce a regrettable compromise in which something very like the infant falling reflex is begun *and resisted*. It is begun unconsciously because of the re-enactment of our earliest reaction to danger. But there is another pattern within us, born, no doubt, of exhortations to 'be brave' – so that, while still very young, we tried not to show fear, perhaps even to ignore it. This acquired behaviour pattern resists the full expression of the reflex – resists it, often, as unconsciously as the reflex was begun. Of course, at a more conscious level, we don't want to react inappropriately to present circumstances and probably don't want our legs to fold up under us! But if and when we become aware of this, both the early and the later patterns are usually already locked in muscular conflict.

In the examples suggested above, the unchecked response to fear could result in breaking something, getting involved in a street accident, making an unfavourable impression, being unfit for fight or flight. The disadvantages, for adults, are obvious. But the usual way of avoiding them produces a contradiction throughout the body, which *tries simultaneously to perform an action and to prevent it* – and this takes its toll of the whole organism.

There is also a 'slow motion' form of the reaction, produced by worry rather than by alarm. Its manifestations are similarly contradictory and similarly hampering. Frequently, there is long-term adaptation to them, which we may even come to accept as normal. Essentially, this adaptation is the typical model of what in this book has been described as *misuse*.[7]

I once made a study of contemporary documents describing health problems of overworked factory hands during the Industrial Revolution in England. One of the most heart-rending things I read was an interview with child workers who did not understand the meaning of the question 'Are you tired?' They had never known what it was like *not* to be tired.[8] I reflected that if this had been the experience of a large section of the population at that time, and if several generations of children had never seen their parents anything but exhausted and bored, and probably worried into the bargain, it was not surprising if they had grown up with poor postural habits.[9] Curiously enough, in the mid-nineteenth century, there was a good deal of awareness of the physical damage that was being done and considerable concern for posterity. It now seems that the damage then done was not hereditary, as was feared at the time – but damage by example is still damage. It is ironic that in our own period there is less fear of 'an enfeebled posterity' than apparently there was in those harsh times. The deterioration that was then feared is now upon us, so that we scarcely notice the familiar patterns of combined collapse and tension, born of fatigue, nurtured by example, sustained by the effects of two world wars, and now aggravated by the worries and frustrations associated with widespread unemployment.

The increasing speed of modern life means also that causes for alarm or anxiety present themselves without enough respite for the muscles to recover, without long enough for the body to 'bounce back' into its natural shape. Even the wish to do something particularly well can imply the fear of not succeeding – and hence can trigger the pattern. When nerves and muscles are trained by repetition in this type of pattern, the habit is reinforced until it becomes difficult not to 'act scared' even when nothing is further from one's mind. This modified infant reflex thus becomes the background to all other activity, a set of unconscious assumptions, the basis for all attempts at co-ordination. We are all in this trap, it seems, with no obvious way out of it.

However, if fear-reactions are part of our genetic inheritance, so also is the solution to the problems they present. An important contribution to our hope of emerging from our plight comes from research that has been done into the 'Startle Pattern': defining it as 'the stereotyped postural response to a loud noise', F.P. Jones refers to it as a 'total reflex'. It seems to me that Startle Pattern, as he shows it in adults, is precisely what I have described above as the contradictory or compromise reaction to the left-over-from-infancy response to the sensation of falling. (Fig. 58, which shows the subject's reaction to the sudden slamming of a door, merits careful study.) *The sequence starts with the change in the relation of head to neck*. Only then, though rapidly, does the pattern take over the rest of the body. Experiments, with stimuli varying from a dropped book to a revolver shot, showed that '*whenever the stimulus was strong enough to elicit a response, it appeared in the neck muscles; in many cases it appeared nowhere else.*'[10]

The good news is that a person who has grasped this fact sufficiently to have integrated it in daily living can often prevent the reaction before it starts. Here is a point where conscious intervention can be helpful. Forewarned is forearmed. Since we know where the sequence begins, we also know where it can be forestalled. It is possible to say 'This situation may become frightening (embarrassing/annoying/whatever) so I shall probably pull my head backwards and downwards unless I now remind myself that my chances will be better if I don't.' This is yet another reason why throughout this book I have emphasized the importance of free balance of the head. (**See especially Chapter 14.**)

This is no mere theorizing on my part; every day of my life confirms the practical significance of these considerations. Moreover, thanks to having thought a lot about the importance of forestalling 'Startle Pattern' in the small events of daily life, I have twice been able to avoid potential motorway accidents. The first time, when I was quite a new driver, had the often-rehearsed thought not instantly flashed through my mind: '*Now* I must not pull my head backwards; *now*, terrified as I am, I need my best co-ordination', the results could have been disastrous, for the typical pattern would have stiffened my arms and legs, interfering with my control of the car; it would also have compromised my view of the road. As it was, hands and feet seemed miraculously to know what to do and the danger passed. I had clearly felt fear trying to take over my whole body but attention to my head-neck relationship had stopped it happening.

Speed of reaction, muscular efficiency, balance, the shape of the framework, the long-term health of joints – all these depend on a good working relationship between the head and the rest of the body. It follows that if 'Startle Pattern' is allowed to get such a hold on us as to become a way of life, all these will suffer.

A good deal of impetus to improvement in this field comes from the performing arts. Surprising? Not at all: the fear of making a fool of oneself is a powerful motive for research in the field of self-management! And musicians, actors, dancers and the like (despite the myth of the artist dreaming away on cloud thirteen) are often practical enough to realize vividly that they depend on their co-ordination to an even greater extent than most other people. They don't always come up with all the answers – who does? But they often have a shrewd idea what the questions are! The performing arts were the ground in which Alexander's discoveries were rooted. The validity of the discoveries has been *recognized* by anatomists, anthropologists, biologists, neurologists, physiologists, psychologists – by the experts; but let us not forget that they were *made*, not by an 'expert' but by an actor, determined to solve a practical problem.

If he could make the discoveries, we can use them. I think we should give ourselves credit for being capable of understanding what we need to know. There is a body of information: this book is my attempt to make it more accessible. As I said in the beginning, this is too important a subject to be left to experts and indeed there is no way of doing so. These are matters in which we all have an interest – and a responsibility.

Although today many people are seeking a better way of using themselves, there is a lack of clarity about what this better way might be. What does it look like, what does it feel like? Despite the efforts of P.E. teachers, ergonomics experts, doctors, physiothera-pists, psychologists, osteopaths and all the other specialists (not to mention the writers of would-be-helpful magazine articles and the steady output of health-and-exercise books, some well-informed, some not) year by year more people suffer from back pain, RSI, breathing difficulties and a whole string of what are called 'stress diseases'.[11]

This is less astonishing than it sounds; we must remember that the experts also are conditioned by the same influences as the rest of us. For by now a modified form of quasi-permanent 'Startle Pattern' is so general that few people question it in themselves or in others. Reactions of the 'Startle' type (fig. 59–75) now look and feel so familiar that they seem 'natural'. Having virtually lost the good examples from whom we could have learnt by semi-conscious imitation (the easiest and most direct form of learning) we need to rediscover consciously what perhaps the human race once knew instinctively.

How can this be achieved? Only by individuals placing themselves face to face with a series of small, private, seemingly insignificant choices. Once we understand and experi-ence the advantages of using ourselves in a more practical way, we ask ourselves more and more often: 'Hold on a moment. Do I want to imitate what I see around me? Is the present problem really a reason to make things even worse for myself? Do I need to pull my head backwards just now?'

It is pleasant to exercise such choices. Presently, too, as a side-benefit, it may happen that our behaviour touches an imitative note in others, perhaps freeing them from some unnecessary discomfort. Usually one can't know this, for talking about it would spoil it – but just occasionally one can guess at what is happening. Of course, the choice must be a real one. It is generally assumed that theoretical knowledge qualifies one to advise other people; the suggestion that one might first question one's own familiar habits is not always welcome. However, no amount of correcting, pretending or 'good posture' will have the same effect as a series of personal decisions genuinely not to do the things that we know are self-destructive.

I think the need for this silent turn-around is one of the biggest challenges facing hu-manity today and one in which we each have a personal part to play, a part that cannot be played by anyone else. Nor can it be played as an intellectual game, for hope lies in the willingness of each individual to reconsider, in practical terms, the assumptions upon which he or she moves through our world.

The epigraph to this chapter is taken from 'The Princess and the Goblin', a favourite book of my childhood which still provides food for thought. In the incident quoted, the little princess was foolish, of course, in a way that we can understand all too well. But having survived to learn from her mistake, she was able to follow a magic thread into the uncharted interior of the mountain, and to come to the help of a young miner who was trapped there.

For me, the magic thread, which leads us through the labyrinth towards freedom, is the use of the head that I have constantly emphasized. It is thanks to past mistakes (my own and other people's) that I have been able to write about it. I hope that what I have learnt may be of help to you.

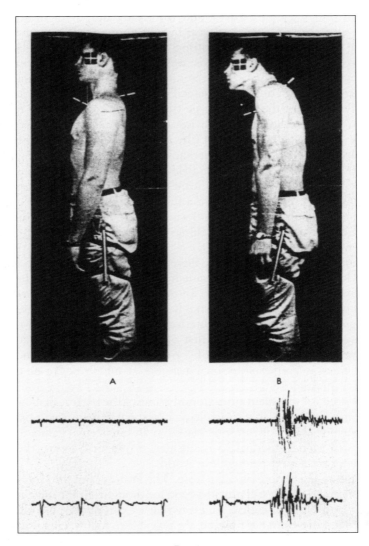

— *Fig. 58* —
Startle pattern
A: 'most comfortable' posture; B: posture after startle stimulus.
Electromyograms of upper trapezius and sternomastoid.

— Figs. 59–75 —

Reactions derived from 'Startle pattern': varying stimuli, same typical disturbance of head-neck region.

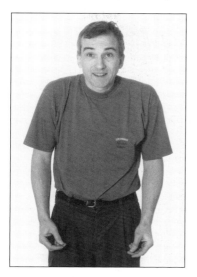

— Fig. 59 —
timidity

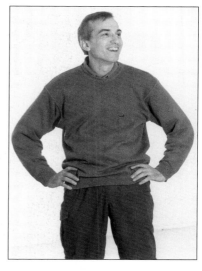

— Fig. 60 —
shyness

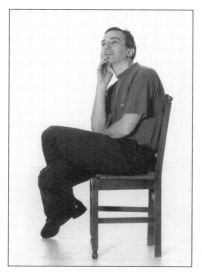

— Fig. 61 —
self-consciousness

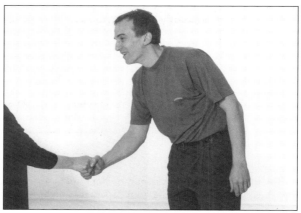

— Fig. 62 —
deference

235

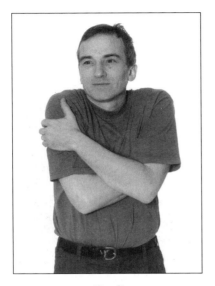

— *Fig. 63* —
cold

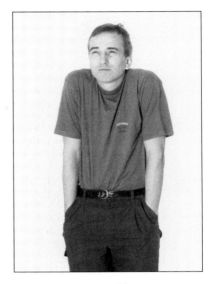

— *Fig. 64* —
dejection

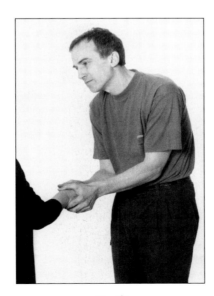

— *Fig. 65* —
sympathy

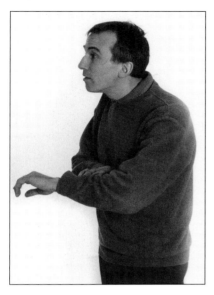

_ *Fig. 66* _
urgency

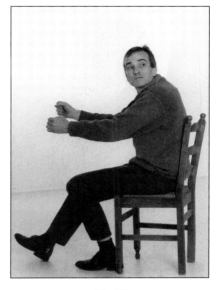

_ *Fig. 67* _
traffic

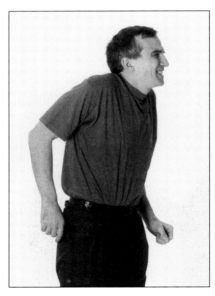

_ *Fig. 68* _
pain

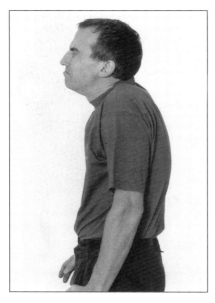

— *Fig. 69* —
breakage

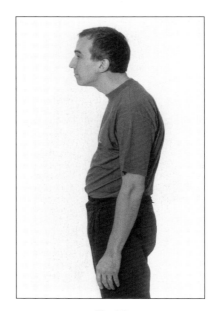

— *Fig. 70* —
defensiveness

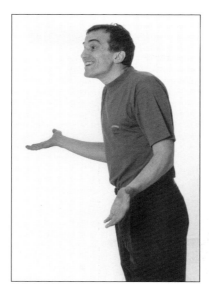

— *Fig. 71* —
excuses

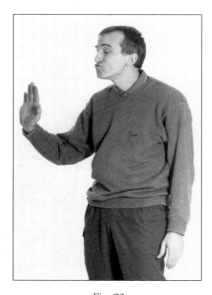

— *Fig. 72* —
argument

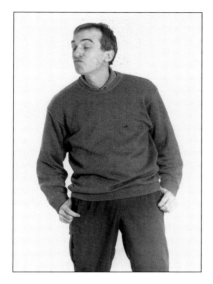

_ *Fig. 73* _
insult

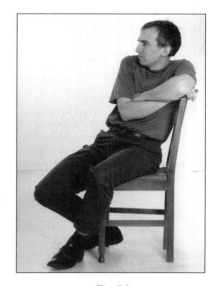

_ *Fig. 74* _
resentment

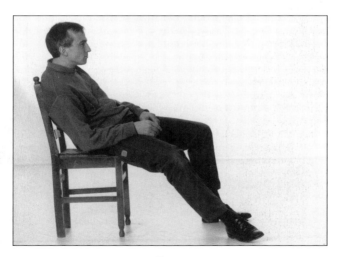

_ *Fig. 75* _
boredom

1. The reaction is composed of several reflexes, which are usually described separately. For present purposes, there are practical reasons for considering them together, e.g. the observation by several authorities that the grasping reflex inhibits the Moro reflex – as one would expect in a real-life situation.
2. E. Vurpillot, in *Grand dictionnaire de la Psychologie*, Paris, Larousse, 1991, p. 479, describes the two phases of the Moro reflex:
   '... first, the arms move sideways away from the body, the back arches and the head is thrown backwards, then the upper limbs return into flexion and adduction...'
   (*'... tout d'abord, les bras s'écartent du corps, le dos s'arque et la tête est rejetée en arrière, puis les membres supérieurs reviennent en flexion et adduction...'*)
3. *ibid.*, p. 24 The grasping reflex is also described as two-part:
   '... in fact, two reflexes or two parts of the same reflex. The first is provoked by stimulation of the palmar side of the fingers. These flex ... and maintain a tight hold on the object touching them. The second is caused by strong pressure on the tendons of the fingers; thus, obviously, it can follow the first ... it is much stronger than the first and can spread to the whole upper limb. Thus the experimenter, placing his finger in the subject's palm, can see the hand tighten around it, and in this way be able to lift the infant's entire body.'
   (*'... en fait, deux réflexes ou deux parties d'un même réflexe. Le premier est provoqué par la stimulation de la face interne des doigts. Ceux-ci fléchissent ... et maintiennent fortement serré l'objet présenté. Le second a pour cause une forte pression sur les tendons des doigts; c'est en ce sens qu'il peut évidemment suivre l'exécution du précédent ... Il est beaucoup plus puissant que le précédent et peut diffuser à tout le membre supérieur. C'est ainsi que l'expérimentateur peut, en présentant un doigt qu'il met dans la main du sujet, voir cette dernière se serrer dessus et soulever ainsi tout le corps de l'enfant...'*)
4. F.M. Feldenkrais, *Body and Mature Behaviour*, London, Routledge and Kegan Paul, 1949, Chapter 10, 'The Body Pattern of Anxiety':
   '... The similarity of reaction of a new-born infant to withdrawal of support, and that of fright or fear in the adult is remarkable. This reaction to falling is present at birth i.e. inborn and independent of individual experience ... no reaction similar to that sensed as fear by the adult can be elicited in the new-born baby, except by sharply altering its position in space...'
5. R.A. Dart, *The postural Aspect of Malocclusion* (1946) reprinted in Dart, *Skill and Poise*, London STAT Books, 1996, p. 79: 'The trapezius ... can operate, quite inappropriately, as an additional retractor (or extensor) of the head.'
   Inappropriate or not, this use of *trapezius* is frequently seen in faulty posture.
6. See also F.P. Kendall and E.K. McCreary, *Muscles – Testing and Function,* Baltimore, Williams and Wilkins, 3rd edition, 1983, p. 117, on shortness of upper trapezius.
7. F.P. Jones, *Freedom to Change*, London, Mouritz, 1997, p. 148:
   'The Startle Pattern may be taken as a paradigm of malposture in general, whether it is associated with aging, disease, or lack of exercise...'
8. Children's Employment Commission's Report, 1843, Commissioner Horne's Report and Evidence, quoted in F. Engels, *The Condition of the Working-Class in England in 1844*, reprinted London, George Allen and Unwin, 1952.
9. R. Roberts, *The Classic Slum*, University of Manchester Press, 1971, reprinted Penguin, 1973, p. 88, includes this reminiscence of growing up in Salford during the first quarter of the twentieth century:
   'Under the common bustle crouched fear. In children – fear of parents, teachers, the Church, the police and authority of any sort; in adults – fear of petty chargehands, foremen, managers and employers of labour ... a dread of sickness, debt, loss of status; above all of losing a job ... Fear was the leitmotif of their lives...'
10. F.P. Jones, *Freedom to Change*, p. 132: 'The change ... begins in the head and neck, passing down the trunk and legs to be completed in about half a second.'
11. Certified absence due to back pain doubled in the 1970s and again in the 1980s; it increased from 59 million days in 1989 to 120 million days in 1996/7. (National Back Pain Association statistics.)

PART VII

DISCOVERING THE MAP

CHAPTER 34

A SHORT ACCOUNT OF THE ALEXANDER TECHNIQUE

> A new experience is like travelling through unknown country. But, remember, others have taken that route before you... So, question number one: is there a map? ... Doesn't matter if you're going to get married, commit a burglary or keep a guinea-pig – efficiency is the proper collation of information.
>
> Alan Bennett *Talking Heads: Soldiering On*

In Australia, in the eighteen-eighties, a young actor, Frederick Matthias Alexander, saw his promising career threatened by chronic hoarseness and frequent loss of voice. He feared the problem might be organic but, although doctors could reassure him on this point, neither they nor his voice teachers could find a solution. Reasoning that, illness having been ruled out, the cause must be technical, he set himself to discover 'what it was that I did that caused the trouble.'

> Without any outside help he worked out, during a series of agonizing years, how to improve what is now called the 'use' of his body musculature in all his postures and movements. And the remarkable outcome was that he regained control of his voice. This story, of perceptiveness, of intelligence, and of persistence, shown by a man without medical training, is one of the true epics of medical research and practice.
> (Professor Nicolaas Tinbergen – Nobel Oration, 1973)

The story has been told many times – but never so well as by Alexander himself in *The Use of the Self*[1] – how he began quite simply to observe himself with the help of mirrors, and noticed that certain changes in the attitude of his head appeared when he started to recite. Going further into the matter, he became aware of other dynamic relationships in the body, which were associated with these unfavourable changes in the relation of head to neck. Finding himself, despite his training in voice and movement, apparently incapable of organizing his body in a way that would permit good functioning of the larynx and breathing apparatus, he came to recognize that vocal quality depends on a total co-ordination in which thought processes are included.

After pursuing his self-imposed line of enquiry and overcoming many discouraging set-backs, Alexander had considerable success as an actor, presenting a one-man show which included excerpts from Shakespeare, and acquiring renown for his voice production and breathing technique. Actors and singers flocked to him for lessons and doctors

243

sent him patients with respiratory problems.

Leading doctors, convinced of the importance of Alexander's discoveries, persuaded him to go to London where they could become more widely known. There, the leading actors of the day (including Sir Henry Irving) became his pupils, as did such writers as G.B. Shaw and Aldous Huxley. (Alexander's influence is present in Huxley's *Eyeless in Gaza* and *Ends and Means*.) Professor John Dewey, philosopher and educationist, also became his pupil and friend: *Human Nature and Conduct* and *Experience and Nature* are impregnated with Alexander's thinking. (In his classic introduction to *The Use of the Self*, Dewey touchingly describes himself as 'from the practical standpoint an inept, awkward and slow pupil'.) The head of the Froebel Institute encouraged Alexander to start a training course for teachers of his technique. The *British Medical Journal* published a letter from nineteen distinguished doctors, exhorting those responsible for medical training to take note of the new field of knowledge opened up by Alexander's discoveries.[2]

There is no lack of witnesses to the importance of these discoveries. George Bernard Shaw wrote:

> He established not only the beginnings of a far reaching science of the apparently involuntary movements we call reflexes, but a technique of correction and self control which forms a substantial addition to our very slender resources in personal education.[3]

Carrington[4] points out that it was only in 1924 that Magnus, writing on the physiology of posture, demonstrated the importance of head/neck reflexes[5] – without proposing any means for making practical use of the information. Alexander's practical technique precedes Magnus by about thirty years.

At a time when problems were classified as either *physical* or *mental*, Alexander had come to the conclusion that each person, each self, is a psychophysical unity, and that *this entire self is inevitably concerned in whatever we happen to be doing*. The concept is not easily expressed: there are plenty of terms that allow us to consider a human being as an ensemble of component parts, but for discussing the whole person, specific language is lacking, as R.D. Laing has pointed out.[6] This lack reflects our habitual way of thinking – but limits the development of our capabilities.

Alexander took as the starting-point for his research the hypothesis that *use affects functioning*. Anyone who has ever said to a child 'Don't muck about with that – you'll spoil it' has obviously grasped the principle in relation to *things*. If today a growing number of people recognize that it is also applicable to *ourselves*, it is chiefly thanks to Alexander. The principle (sometimes called 'the Alexander Principle') was merely a starting-point. How could he make practical use of it?

Several stages were needed. First came a long period of *observation*, during which obstacles were identified and Alexander came to realize that secure voice functioning depends on the total co-ordination. Therefore he sought a *means* of erecting what one might describe as a scaffolding of conditions that would favour the healthy use of his voice; a means whereby he could establish and maintain this 'scaffolding' during vocal work and throughout the multitude of activities one might ask of the human organism.

Alexander discovered the means he was seeking, in the fact that certain dynamic relationships within the body (notably, but not exclusively, that of the head to the vertebral column) influence the functioning of the rest of the organism. He described the ensemble of these relationships as constituting the primary control of the use of himself in all his activities, *a primary control of the general use of the self.*[7] The term 'primary control' has been subject to misinterpretation and controversy, but as Professor F.P. Jones has pointed out,[8] the arguments are merely verbal; in practice, there is no room for doubt about the validity of Alexander's teaching on this point. This *is what happens;* nature has provided each of us with a 'primary control' – how we use it is what Alexander's work was all about. In corroboration, the neurologist Sherrington wrote:

> Mr Alexander has done a service to the subject by insistently treating each act as involving the whole integrated individual, the whole psycho-physical man. To take a step is an affair, not of this or that limb solely, but of the total neuromuscular activity of the moment – not least of the head and neck.[9]

The search for means entered upon a second stage when a major difficulty emerged: humanity is endowed by nature with innumerable possibilities of movement, which can also give rise to innumerable possibilities of confusion. More often than we know, we try to make, simultaneously, movements that are mutually contradictory. Worse still, we tend to construct habits based on these contradictions, and to assume that the associated kinaesthetic sensations are 'right' and 'normal'. Happily, nature has also provided a means of avoiding unhelpful movements in favour of more efficient ones. Sherrington explained that '... to refrain from an act is no less an act than to commit one, because inhibition is co-equally with excitation a nervous activity.'[10] More recently, Changeux proposed that *'apprendre, c'est éliminer'*[11] and Libet has drawn attention to the part played by inhibition in neurological aspects of decision making.[12]

In current usage, this word *inhibition* has acquired a very different connotation from its literal neurological meaning.[13] In fact, without inhibition (in the exact sense) *excitation* could affect any muscle, leading to anarchy in movement. Inhibition, therefore, is a fundamental function of the nervous system and much of our reflex functioning depends on it. We all use it unconsciously. However, certain people make more use of inhibition than others: a skilful person is one who performs desired actions without adding useless efforts. It is in this sense that we should understand Alexander's 'conscious inhibition', the purpose of which is to widen the area of free choice. It precedes the organization of the basic co-ordination, which in turn should precede the aiming of our energies at a specific end.

Conscious inhibition paves the way for ***direction***, the third step of Alexander's reasoned means whereby satisfactory co-ordination can be achieved. The word 'direction' here implies all the usual meanings, as in 'over there', 'directions for use' and 'orchestra under the direction of...'. Alexander explains that he uses the term 'to indicate the process involved in projecting messages from the brain to the mechanisms and in conducting the energy necessary to the use of these mechanisms.'[14]

The combination of inhibition and direction erects the scaffolding and prepares the quality of the desired movement. By liberating us from habits that may be useless or even harmful, inhibition and direction clear a path for the action of our reflexes – and relieve us of too great a preoccupation with the details of our 'posture' and of our actions. Voluntary and reflex elements become better integrated. I am aware that readers unacquainted with the Alexander Technique may feel frustrated by the limited amount of information I have given on these two key concepts of inhibition and direction, but I cannot commit to words the subtle experiences involved in practical learning.

The Alexander approach differs fundamentally from relaxation methods. In fact, the 'relaxation' concept requires cautious handling, for the instruction to relax implies a previous undesirable contraction. The purpose of the inhibition/direction combination is to avoid the parasite contraction *before it occurs* – a factor that is sadly lacking in most forms of education and training. (The ease of skilled persons is admired, while effort *as such* is considered praiseworthy – an absurd contradiction which often goes unrecognized.) Alexander emphasizes that the inhibition of unnecessary reactions offers a reasoned means of aiming our abilities in the direction of our ends. The effort involved (whether it be minute or tremendous, according to the situation) will thus be appropriate to the chosen action.

In solving his own problem, Alexander had made a discovery applicable to every form of human activity. He did not stop there. Having realized that verbal explanation is inevitably understood in terms of the hearer's previous experience, he developed a *teaching technique* which makes use of subtle and precise touch where words might be misleading. The efficiency of the guiding touch depends on the teacher's own co-ordination; there is no question of being able to teach Alexander's discoveries without having integrated them into one's own daily life. Consequently the training of Alexander teachers demands a great deal of individual attention to the co-ordination of each trainee, during a minimum of three years. There is cause for concern when, for instance, physiotherapists claim to 'practise the Alexander technique' (*sic*) as an adjunct to treatments they offer. The Society of Teachers of the Alexander Technique (STAT) has been in existence since 1958 and can be regarded as an authority on the requirements for teaching the Alexander Technique. The special skills developed by the aspiring Alexander teacher are profoundly different from the physiotherapist's approach. But only those few physiotherapists with a diploma in Alexander teaching will be able to appreciate this, since it is only after the three years of training that the need for those three years is fully understood.

To sum up: the Alexander Technique is not a postural technique as such; indeed, Alexander is quoted as saying, 'There is no such thing as a right position, but there is such a thing as a right direction.' It is not concerned with relaxation, massage or manipulation; nor is it a series of exercises. (An exercise may be good or bad according to the co-ordination of the person who performs it.) By learning progressively to abandon useless habits, and thanks to a continuous reflex adaptation of the balance between tension and relaxation, the pupil discovers postures and ways of moving that are more natural and better suited to the demands of each activity. The same basic principles can be applied to the most ordinary of everyday acts, as well as to the more complex requirements of music, dance or sport. These same principles assist doctors and psychologists in their observation of patients, since knowing the 'directions for use' that the patient has given himself can be an important element in diagnosis.

It would be idle to pretend that an Alexander teacher is a standard product, any more than a tennis player, a pianist or a doctor. As in any profession, some practitioners are more experienced than others, some are more gifted, some have been better trained. Among Alexander teachers can be found those who rely chiefly on touch as a method of communication, whereas others enjoy responding to requests for verbal explanation. Some are particularly fascinated by the application of the Technique to specific skills in which they are themselves expert, while others prefer to concern themselves with fundamentals. In practice, things are rarely as cut-and-dried as this may seem to imply. (Two other approaches should, in my opinion, be viewed with caution. It is possible to become too eclectic, and thus to risk diluting Alexander's message with ideas borrowed from elsewhere; on the other hand, where a teacher's outlook is unduly restricted, the Technique may be reduced to a conditioning process, in which the same phrases are repeated in the hope that they will eventually acquire meaning for the pupil.) As each pupil is different, so does each teacher bring to his or her work a particular experience of life, and special knowledge and talents. Naturally therefore, it can happen that one pupil will not get on well with a certain teacher, but the right teacher can usually be found. Beyond all individual variations, Alexander offers us basic principles, universal and unchanging, which one cannot afford to ignore, for they govern the human organism in all its activities.

---

1. F.M. Alexander, *The Use of the Self*, London, Gollancz, 1996, Chapter 1.
2. *British Medical Journal*, 29th May, 1937, letter signed by nineteen doctors:
   '... We are convinced that Alexander is justified in contending that "an unsatisfactory manner of use, by interfering with general functioning, constitutes a predisposing cause of disorder and disease" and that diagnosis ... must remain incomplete unless ... (it) takes into consideration the influence of use upon functioning.'
3. G.B. Shaw (1937), *Shaw's Music*, London, Bodley Head, 1981, Vol.1, p. 46.
4. W. Carrington and S. Carey, *Walter Carrington on the Alexander Technique*, London, Sheildrake, 1986, p. 38.
5. R. Magnus, *Körperstellung*, Berlin, Springer, 1924.
6. R.D. Laing, *The Divided Self*, Harmondsworth, Penguin (Pelican), 1965, pp. 19–20:
   'The most serious objection to the vocabulary currently used ... is that it consists of words which split man up verbally ... we cannot give an adequate account of the existential splits unless we can begin from the concept of a unitary whole, and no such concept exists, nor can any such concept be expressed within the current language system ... we have an already shattered Humpty Dumpty who cannot be put together again by any number of ... compound words: psycho-physical, psycho-somatic, psycho-social, etc.'
7. F.M. Alexander, *op. cit.* The original edition (Methuen, 1932) has (Chapter 1):
   '... in short, that to lengthen *I must put my head forward and up. As is shown by what follows, this proved to be the primary control of my use in all my activities.*'
   The 1946 edition (Integral Press) after '... forward and up' continues:
   '*The experiences which followed my awareness of this were forerunners of a recognition of that relativity in the use of the head, neck, and other parts which proved to be a primary control of the general use of the self.*'
   The 1985 Gollancz edition reverts to the 1932 text. The omission seems a matter for regret. It can, of course, be argued that surrounding paragraphs already make it plain that misuse of the head is 'inseparably bound up with a misuse of other mechanisms'. Yet Alexander apparently found it desirable to clarify this mention of the all-important primary control.

8. F.P. Jones, *Freedom to Change*, London, Mouritz, 1997, p. 48:
'Some doctors objected to the comparison of Alexander's primary control with the central control (*Zentralapparat*) of Magnus on the grounds that Magnus was referring not to the relation of head to trunk but to the anatomical center in the brainstem where the postural reflexes are integrated. This is a verbal quibble. Alexander did not claim to have discovered an anatomical center; Magnus, on the other hand, did not rest his explanation on the location of the center but on the function of the reflexes. The doctrine of a 'primary control', whether or not it was the same one as demonstrated by Magnus, provided Alexander with a parsimonious explanation for his findings ... The term was accepted by Dewey and by most of the medical men who wrote about the Technique in the twenties and thirties ... Ludovici, whose information came from the Körperstellung itself ... assembled a large number of passages from both Magnus and Sherrington to show the bearing of their work on Alexander's.'
9. C. Sherrington, *The Endeavour of Jean Fernel*, Cambridge University Press, 1946, p. 89.
10. C. Sherrington, *The Brain and its Mechanism* (see above, Chapter 10, note 2.).
11. J.P. Changeux, *L'Homme Neuronal*, Fayard, 1983, p. 326.
12. B. Libet, 'Unconscious cerebral initiative and the role of conscious will in voluntary action', in *The Behavioural and Brain Sciences*, 1985, 8, 529:
'I propose the thesis that conscious volitional control may operate not to initiate the volitional process but to select and control it, either by permitting or triggering the final motor outcome of the consciously initiated process or by vetoing the progression to actual motor activation.'
13. For definition of *inhibition*, see above, Chapter 10, Note 3.
14. F.M. Alexander, *op. cit.* p. 35, footnote.

SUGGESTED FURTHER READING ABOUT
THE ALEXANDER TECHNIQUE

From the considerable amount that has been written on the subject (STAT Books has the most comprehensive list) I have chosen only books that are readily available and that I can recommend as useful to newcomers to the Alexander Technique. All are available from STAT Books, 20, London House, 266 Fulham Rd, London SW10 9EL
Tel: +44 171 352 0666, E-mail: stat@pavilion.co.uk

The Use of the Self
F.M. Alexander (1932) Gollancz, 1985, ISBN 0 575 03720 2
The third, shortest and most approachable of Alexander's four books, describing how he made his original discovery and exploring some of the implications.

Explaining the Alexander Technique
Walter Carrington in conversation with Seán Carey, Sheildrake, 1992,
ISBN 0 951998 8 X
The essential companion to Alexander's works. Alexander's principal assistant answers questions posed by an anthropologist who is himself a teacher of the Alexander Technique: the fruit of nearly sixty years' thinking about and around the subject, clear and readable.

Body Learning
Michael Gelb, Aurum, 1981, 1987, 1994, ISBN 1 85410 286 9
This expanded version of a degree thesis makes a good introduction to the Alexander Technique; enhanced by well-chosen photographs.

BIBLIOGRAPHY

Alexander, F.M. *The Theory and Practice of a New Method of Respiratory Re-education* (1907) reprinted in
   F.M. Alexander *Articles and Lectures*, London, Mouritz, 1995
Alexander, F.M. *The Use of the Self*, London, Gollancz, 1996
Alexander, F.M. *Constructive Conscious Control of the Individual* (1923) London, STAT Books, 1997
Basmajian, J.V. *Primary Anatomy*, Baltimore, Williams and Wilkins, 7th edition, 1976
Bloom, Anthony (Archbishop) *Living Prayer*, London, Darton, Longman and Todd, 1966
Bonnier, P. *La Voix – sa culture physiologique*, Paris, Alcan, 1910
Carrington, W. and Carey, S. *Walter Carrington on the Alexander Technique*, London, Sheildrake, 1986
Carrington, W. and Carey, S. *Explaining the Alexander Technique*, London, Sheildrake, 1992
Cerutty, Percy Wells *Athletics – how to become a champion*, London, Stanley Paul, 1960
Changeux, J.P. *L'Homme Neuronal*, Fayard, 1983
Chariton, Igumen of Valamo *The Art of Prayer – an Orthodox Anthology*, London, Faber and Faber, 1966
Children's Employment Commission's Report, 1843, Commissioner Horne's Report and Evidence, quoted
   in F. Engels *The Condition of the Working-Class in England in 1844*, reprinted London, George Allen and
   Unwin, 1952
Dart, R.A. *The Postural Aspect of Malocclusion* (1946) reprinted in Dart, *Skill and Poise*, London, STAT
   Books, 1996
Dart, R.A. *The Attainment of Poise* (1947) reprinted in Dart, *Skill and Poise*, London, STAT Books, 1996
Dart, R.A. 'Voluntary musculature in the human body: the double-spiral arrangement', in *British Journal of
   Physical Medicine*, 1950, reprinted in Dart, *Skill and Poise*, London, STAT Books, 1996
Dewey, J. *Human Nature and Conduct (an introduction to social psychology)* New York, Holt, 1922
Dürckheim, K. von *The Japanese Cult of Tranquillity*, transl. E. O'Shiel, London, Rider, 1960
Feldenkrais, M. *Body and Mature Behaviour*, London, Routledge and Kegan Paul, 1949
Gorman, David 'In our own image', in *Alexander Review*, 1987, vol. 2, no.1
Gray's *Anatomy*, Longman, Edinburgh, 35th edition, 1973
Gurdjieff, G. I. *Views from the Real World*, Dutton, 1973
Hazrat Inayat Khan *The Music of Life*, New York, Omega, 1983
Husler, F. and Rodd-Marling, Y. *Singing: the physical nature of the vocal organ*, London, Hutchinson, revised
   edition, 1976
Jones, F.P. 'Method for changing stereotyped response patterns by the inhibition of certain postural sets', in
   Psychological Review, 1965, 72, 196/214
Jones, F.P. *Freedom to Change*, London, Mouritz, 1997
Kapandji, I.A. *The Physiology of the Joints*, Edinburgh, Churchill Livingstone, 1974
Kendall, F.P. and McCreary, E.K. *Muscles – Testing and Function*, Baltimore, Williams and Wilkins, 3rd edi-
   tion, 1983
Laing, R.D. *The Divided Self*, Harmondsworth, Penguin (Pelican), 1965
Libet, 'Unconscious cerebral initiative and the role of conscious will in voluntary action', in *The Behavioural
   and Brain Sciences*, 1985, 8, 529

Magnus, R. 'Some results of studies in the physiology of posture' (Cameron Prize Lectures), in *Lancet*, 1926, Sept. 11

Magnus, R. *Körperstellung*, Berlin, Springer, 1924

Maslow, A. *The Farther Reaches of Human Nature*, Harmondsworth, Penguin (Pelican) 1973

Ouspensky, P.D. *In Search of the Miraculous*, London, Routledge and Kegan Paul, 1950

Pantañjali *How to know God – the Yoga aphorisms of Pantañjali*, transl. Swami Pravhavananda and C. Isherwood, Signet, 1969

Platzer, W. *Color Atlas and Textbook of Human Anatomy, vol. 1, Locomotor System*, New York, Thieme, 4th English edition, 1992

Roberts, R. *The Classic Slum*, University of Manchester Press, 1971, reprinted Penguin, 1973

Roberts, T.D.M. *Understanding Balance*, London, Chapman and Hall, 1995

Sears, W.G. *Anatomy and Physiology for Nurses and Students of Human Biology*, London, Edward Arnold, 4th edition, 1965

Shaw, G.B. (1937) *Shaw's Music*, London, Bodley Head, 1981, Vol.1

Sherrington, C. *The Brain and its Mechanism*, Rede Lecture, Cambridge University, (C.U.P.), 1933 quoted in *Selected Writings of Sir Charles Sherrington*, ed. D. Denny-Brown, Oxford University Press, 1979

Sherrington, C. *Man on his Nature*, Cambridge University Press, 1940

Sherrington, C. *The Endeavour of Jean Fernel*, Cambridge University Press, 1946

Struyf-Denys, G. *Les Chaînes musculaires et articulaires,* Société Belge d'Ostéopathie et de Recherche en Thérapie Manuelle, 1978

Taisen Deshimaru *Zen et Arts Martiaux*, Paris, Seghers, 1977

The Bulletin – the newsweekly of the capital of Europe, Brussels, 21st November, 1996

The Independent, 14th June, 1995

Vurpillot, E. in *Grand dictionnaire de la Psychologie*, Paris, Larousse, 1991

For further information about the Alexander Technique, contact the Society of Teachers of the Alexander Technique (STAT) or one of its affiliated societies.

STAT was established in 1958 with the aims of maintaining and improving professional standards; making the Technique more widely known; facilitating contact between members; encouraging research into the Technique; preventing abuse and exploitation by untrained people. All members on the teaching lists have completed a full-time three year training course. A programme of post-graduate education and training is provided for members. Members are bound by a Code of Professional Conduct. STAT has acted as an advisory body for the formation of similar national organizations outside the UK.

Addresses

The Society of Teachers of the Alexander Technique (STAT), 129 Camden Mews – London NW1 9AH
Tel: +44 207 482 5135 – Fax: +44 207 482 5435
e-mail: office@stat.org.uk – website: http://www.stat.org.uk

STAT-affiliated societies:

Australia	**AUSTAT**, Australian Society of Teachers of the A.T. PO Box 716, Darlinghurst, NSW 2010. Tel.: 008 339 571
Belgium	**AEFMAT**, 4 rue des Fonds, 1380 Lasne Tel/fax: 02/633 3059
Brazil	**ABTA**, Rua dos Miranhas, 333, cep: 05434-040, Sao Paulo-SP
Canada	**CANSTAT**, 1472 E.St.Joseph Bvd., Apt.No.4, Montreal, Quebec, H2J 1M5. Tel: 514 522 9230
Denmark	**DFLAT**, Amager Faelledvej 4, DK-2300 Copenhagen S Tel: 32 96 20 19 – Fax: 32 96 20 39
France	**APTA**, 42, Terrasse de l'Iris, La Défense 2, 92400 Courbevoie Fax: 0140 90 06 23
Germany	**GLAT**, Postfach 5312, 79020 Freiburg. Tel: 0761 383357
Israel	**ISTAT**, PO Box 715, Karkur 37106. Tel: 06 378244
Netherlands	**NeVLAT**, Postbus 15591, 1001 NB Amsterdam. Tel: 020 625 3163
South Africa	**SASTAT**, 5,Leinster Road, Green Point 8001. Tel: 021 439 3440
Spain	**APTAE**, 156 AP, 28080 Madrid
Switzerland	**SVLAT**, Postfach, CH-8032 Zurich. Tel: 01 201 0343
USA	**AMSAT**, 401 East Market Street, Charlottesville VA 22902 Tel: 804 295 2480 – Fax: 804 295 3947

Austria has a STAT-approved teacher training course. For details of this, and of Alexander teachers in Antigua, Argentina, Austria, Bulgaria, Colombia, Eire, Hong Kong, India, Italy, Japan, Luxembourg, Malaysia, Mexico, New Zealand, Norway, Philippines, Poland, Sweden, Uraguay, contact STAT itself (address above) or your local STAT-affiliated society.